REVIVING THE HEART OF MEDICINE

Emily Anne Sander, MD
Reviving the Heart of Medicine

—

Published by - Spines
ISBN: 979-8-89691-357-3

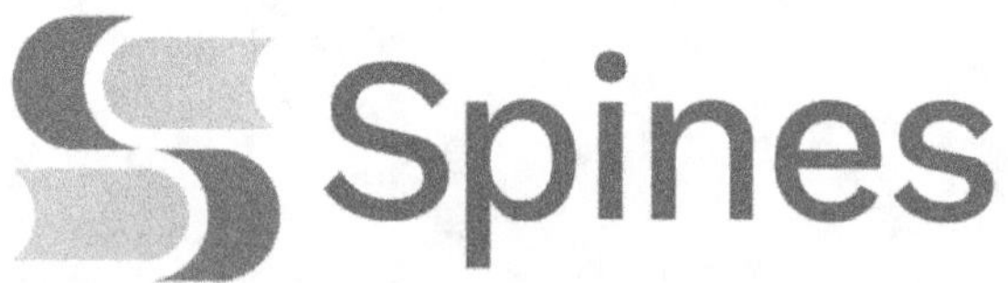

Reviving the Heart of Medicine

Emily Anne Sander, MD

CONTENTS

DEDICATION

This book is dedicated to you.
To all those who pick up this book, thank you for giving my words a chance to be part of your story.
You were created to be healed and whole. To not settle for mediocrity. To know that you are truly loved by the Author of your life. The Creator of your heart.
It is no accident that you have found this book, as its message was placed on my heart to share it with you.
I am forever grateful to my parents, who were the first to plant the seed of the love of God in my heart. Love that would grow despite all hardships. Your example, love and support have made me who I am today.
For my husband, who always believes in me and pushes me to continually reach for more. You are my greatest supporter and the love of my life.
To my daughter Gracie and my children yet to come. You fill me with joy and show me God's goodness every day.
For my mentors who never gave up on me. You know who you

are. The ones who spent countless hours sharing their knowledge with this small-town girl.

To the Women at The Well. Your courage to step out into the unknown with me, and your dedication to care for our patients inspires me daily.

To those no longer with us, Dr. B and Samuel Alexander. Your light still shines to this day. You are forever part of my story and you impact how I practice the art of healing.

To my Savior and King, Jesus Christ. The One who deserves all glory. Let my words reflect a portion of your abundant love. One day with you is better than a thousand elsewhere.

"My flesh and my heart may fail, but God is the strength of my heart and my portion forever."
Psalms 73:26 NIV

FOREWORD

'*Primum non nocere*' – first, do no harm. The solemn oath repeated by all graduates of medical school is attributed to the Greek physician and philosopher Hippocrates and is well known as the eponymous Hippocratic oath. While the importance of such an oath is self-evident, there exist other words spoken by Hippocrates that reflect his wisdom and understanding of what the true meaning of healing encompasses. Words such as, *"Wherever the art of medicine is loved, there is also the love of humanity,"* or *"It is far more important to know what person the disease has than what disease the person has,"* as well as *"The life so short, the craft so long to learn."* Truer words have seldom been spoken, the foundational bedrock of philosophical extrapolation pertaining to the art of medicine never so concisely uttered. Yet, all these sacred tenets have been questioned, derided, altered, and ultimately discarded. In basic terms, medicine in the United States is broken.

Of the thirty-seven miracles attributed to Jesus recorded

in the Gospels, twenty-eight pertain to the healing of a malady or the raising of the dead. What message should we ascertain from such an example? Interestingly, in many cases, the healing was of a non-believer. The Son of God had within his power the ability to awe the world with spectacular supernatural feats, yet he chose to minister the directive of Heaven to render aid to those suffering and in need. The act of healing one's physical ailments opens the gateway to spiritual healing, a fact not lost in Jesus's ministry; however, this fact has all but vanished in modern medicine. The chasm between physical and spiritual healing in modern medical practices has become so deep and wide that it is not only shunned but censored. There are some institutions where one cannot even speak of their personal beliefs for fear that they might possibly offend another. Are one's beliefs so superficially held that another's words can so easily whisk them away? How can free speech not exist in a field where ideas and hypotheses must be challenged every single day?

So, it begins. *The desire to help others* has become a cliché in admission interviews for applicants of medical school, replaced by drills in logical critical thinking. The desired outcome is to produce a medical professional that is able to systematically follow algorithms established under the nomenclature of "standard of care protocol." While this is desirable in most, but not all, hospital settings, the carry-over into office encounters has not only dehumanized the *"Art of Medicine"* but minimizes the importance of patient bonding, establishment of trust, and, in some cases, the diminishment of hope. The logic behind such training falls under the false pretense of efficiency or so it would seem. Proper communication takes time, and in many cases, barriers must be breached to get accurate information from the scared and apprehensive patient, without which medicine becomes based on cursory vital signs and assumptions. The result is often missed or inaccurate diagnosis, over or under-medicating, and poor communication with other members of the patient's healthcare team. Is it any wonder why adverse drug reactions are the fourth leading cause of death in the United States?

Whether in the hospital setting or in the office setting, doctors find themselves faced with the dichotomy of excellent patient care versus the economics of the business of medicine. The annual 1.6 trillion-dollar healthcare industry has adopted a *"one-size-fits-all"* mentality for reimbursements across the board. This disconnect between the actual time needed to provide excellent, individualized care and the ability to keep the lights on must somehow be reconciled by the physician or the institution for whom they are employed. Meanwhile, the average salary for the CEO of insurance companies is more than twenty million dollars annually. In addition, the average cost of insurance coverage for a family of four is north of twenty-five thousand dollars annually, and for that premium, the patients will still receive a bill that may be ruinous.

The complexity of patients' medical problems in the United States may be the only factor rising faster than the cost of care to ameliorate these complex maladies. The increasingly toxic burden from food, air, water, medicines, and the environment has negative effects on individuals daily. It creates massive stress at the cellular level, which not only complicates known diseases but also creates a plethora of new ones. Dealing with such issues on a preventative level seems elementally intuitive; however, the training in most medical schools may comprise a meager one to four hours out of a four-year program, almost as if it were more profitable to allow these conditions rather than prevent them. Physicians being ill-prepared or under-tooled to deal with chronic complex illnesses results in a vicious cycle of medications or treatments used that never address the underlying cause, which leads to more medications to deal with the side effects of the first salvo. All the while, there is the stark realization that, although the patient may feel better, they are, in fact, not getting better, let alone free from disease.

There comes a turning point in everyone's life, and this is true of most healthcare professionals, where introspective analysis occurs, and one questions meaning and purpose. For some, it comes later and for some, it comes early, but rest assured, it does come. Unfortunately, many in the healthcare industry find the answers to be most disagreeable and somewhat depressing. This translates into burnout, diminished self-worth, and frightening cognitive dissonance. Once the realization sinks in that what and where they are usurps the visions, hopes and dreams that led them to enter the field, it makes the person unrecognizable to their inner self. Bringing this all-too-common scenario into focus is the sobering statistics found in a 2024 article in the Journal of Primary Care and Community Health by Jain et al., which states that suicide risk amongst male physicians is 70% higher and females 250% to 400% higher compared to their nonmedical counterparts. Each year, 300-400 physicians commit suicide. The question must be asked: in a profession predicated on humanity and dedicated to improving the welfare of others, how can this be?

Enter the coping mechanisms. For some healthcare workers, coping mechanisms such as alcohol or drug abuse seem to numb the pain, while others spiral into chronic illness or develop a frank mental condition. The catalysts are pressure, long hours, the adaptation to the mindset of being a perfectionist, inculcation in stoicism and diminished colleague interaction and support. Most commonly, there is a recalibration of one's moral compass. Instead of being grounded on the basis of personal standards, convictions and beliefs, slippage begins to undermine those principles. Acceptance of the status quo becomes the norm. After all, it is much easier to go along to get along, all the while fueling the cognitive dissonance. This phenomenon was best illustrated during the COVID pandemic, where doctors were sanctioned, fired and in some cases, stripped of their privileges or license for thinking outside the establishment's protocol, even though it was not working, and doctors knew it. The generation of a new, creative coping mechanism was the participation of doctors and nurses in choreographed dancing, which was posted on the social media platform Tik Tok. This is sadly and egregiously analogous to Nero fiddling while Rome was burning. Thus is the state of medicine.

In the following pages, you will read about one doctor who reached the turning point of self-analysis, weighed the reality of what she saw and found her satisfaction and sense of purpose to be wanting. She never recalibrated her moral compass, nor did she embark on the dependency of coping mechanisms. Instead, she bravely strapped on the armor of God, stayed the course and set her sails for a new direction. She was armed with three powerful allies: courage, perseverance, and faith, all of which were tried and assaulted, but nonetheless, arose victorious. You are about to share memoirs and proverbs ascertained along her journey. Ultimately, she invites you to become one of the many healthcare providers dedicated to bringing humanity and God-based spiritual healing back into the sacred art of medicine. Just as Jesus's final directive to his disciples was to go out into the world and heal the sick, cast out demons, and preach the gospel, a God-centered movement into medicine has begun. Dr. Emily Sander is inviting you to be part of that movement. It won't be easy, nor can you travel this journey alone. However, first and foremost, in the words of Jesus, recorded in the one gospel written by a physician, which is more applicable today than ever before. Physician, heal thyself. Luke 4:23*KJV*

~Harold Landis, DDS, Fellow Integrative Medicine

PREFACE

"Clearly, you are a letter from Christ showing the result of our ministry among you. This "letter" is written not with pen and ink, but with the Spirit of the living God. It is carved not on tablets of stone, but on human hearts."
2 Corinthians 3:3 *NLT*

A book was once given to me, followed by a word. I did not know it then, but it was a book and a word that shifted my world.

That's the thing about words. They are seeds.

They are never meant to lay dormant. Unwatered. Left in the dark.

No, they are always meant to be planted in good soil, to take root and to grow.

Your life is that seed.

It is an open book to those around you. As Paul eloquently spoke, "Written not with pen and ink, but with the Spirit of the living God."

Some of your chapters may be bad, and others will be good, but they are all part of your story. Don't be discouraged if your last one didn't turn out as you wanted.

It is never too late to start a new chapter. Your story is still in the process of being written.

One day, you will look back and realize there are times you may have stumbled or even fallen, but the overall path you were following was taking you closer toward an eternal treasure.

During this journey, you must know that your book and your words are never hidden. Your life story is one that others are currently reading. So, let them read your story. Let them take it in. Let them look forward to the parts that are still unwritten. Let them find treasure in the midst.

Focus on living your life in a way that your book transforms those around you. Let the story of your life lead them to their Author.

Most importantly, let your actions and words shift their atmosphere as the testimony of your life focuses their eyes on Him.

Introduction

"Behold, I will do a new thing; now it shall spring forth; shall ye not know it? I will even make a way in the wilderness and rivers in the desert."
Isaiah 43:19 *ESV*

A Shaking

The fault lines are shaking. Do you feel the movement under your feet? What started out subtle is growing stronger and louder with more turbulence than you expected. What could this be?

You are experiencing a shaking.

A moment where you will look back on one day and sense the seismic shift of the encounter. A moment where you find yourself standing at the fault lines and feel the tremors. These are the kinds of moments that you realize days, months, or maybe years later were always going to be part of your story, yet you did not see them coming.

We begin our journey together in one of these moments.

A moment that still impacts me to this day. One of many I will share with you in this book. Moments of shaking where God's presence tears the veil and we feel His presence, we see His movement, and we hear His voice.

Moments of shaking that change who we are.

My Shaking

Looking back, it was the day I was given a book by a friend that my world really began shaking. It was a day that things began to break apart in the greatest of ways.

It was the early afternoon when my late friend, Dr. B., stopped by to visit me during a shift in the Emergency Department. It was a rare shift where I had a few moments of peace, time to breathe and time to actually catch up with a friend. If you were someone who knew me when I was working in the Emergency Department, you would know how fleeting those moments truly were. Nevertheless, it was a rare moment and one that I would later determine to be a pivotal point in my journey.

It was on that day when I was enjoying a quiet moment in the normally hustling department when I saw him. Dr. B had just come back from some time off and decided to drop by and give me a gift. As I looked up from the provider's desk, I saw a small book in his hands titled The Alchemist by Paulo Coelho.

My friend was very focused when he began talking to me about the book. More serious than I was used to seeing him. He seemed nervous as he was sharing something vulnerable, yet I could sense that he knew he was supposed to share it. He went on. He said the book had opened his eyes to view his life in a new way. It had helped him on his own personal journey of discovering who he was and what he was called to do. He shared that he thought it would be important for me and my journey as well. After we chatted a bit more, he turned around and left as quickly as he had come in.

I chuckled and put the book in my bag, but my curiosity was piqued. What was I about to learn? Hopefully, my shift will pass quickly enough, and I will find the answer to this question.

Although I didn't realize I was standing on a fault line that day, I felt a shift. I sensed the tremors. There was a message I was about to learn. What I didn't comprehend though, was that was the last day I would see my friend alive. That's the thing with moments. We never know how many we will have. We never know when our time is up.

As 5:30 pm rolled around, I quickly signed over my patients to the oncoming physician. I was more than happy to be done for the day. I went home, grabbed a quick snack and began to devour the pages of the book he had given me. I was captivated by the story of the fictional protagonist, Santiago.

As I read on, I learned more about this boy who went on a journey for great treasure, his Personal Legend. As I continued, I learned of a journey that was complicated by many twists and turns. Dr. B was right. It was fantastic.

I loved reading about the unique people he met along the way and the key lessons he learned. But it was the end of his story that got me. It was the end where you saw beauty in his journey. It was in the end that his world was shaken. It was in the final hours of his journey that Santiago learned he could shift the atmosphere around him.

Bright Lights

Reading this book opened my eyes to the knowledge that there are people who will come across our path, even for a short time, who will leave a lasting impact on our destiny. Ones who shift atmospheres. Ones God uses to shake us.

Dr. B was one of those people in my story. God used him to shift my path. A bright light that glimmered only for a moment but whose light still impacts me and how I practice medicine today.

What about you? Who is that bright light in your story? Who are the people who shifted your atmosphere? Who nudged you into your destiny?

When the Ink Hits its Mark

Looking back now, I realized that my friend had brought me that book after months of sharing my messages with him. It was during the dark days of the pandemic when I began writing messages of hope and sending them to friends and family. Messages of encouragement. Messages of God's love. Messages that were placed on my heart.

I didn't realize it as I wrote, but these messages met others in their times of need. When they were going through their own dark times. These messages planted seeds. As I wrote, I spoke words that were placed on my heart. I truly didn't know if they would impact anyone else reading them. I wrote them mostly to encourage myself, but for Dr. B, the messages were more than timely. They were pivotal.

That's the thing with words. We often know it is important to write them but often don't realize what lasting impact they will have. We don't always see what happens when the ink hits its mark.

Knowing now the end of my friend's story, I am forever thankful that I followed through and sent those messages. My messages to my friend were of God's love. They were simple, but they were effective. My friend's final message to me was about seeking treasure that, in the end, happened to be learning to shift the atmosphere. Messages that were separate but in the end, related.

That's the thing with words. Everyone's messages are unique. They are part of a bigger picture, part of a tapestry woven together. Your words matter. Your story matters. Never think that He won't use you or your story.

God will use your words to speak to those around you. If you let Him, He will use you as a good seed.

Imagine what messages you are being called to write or speak today that could make all the difference to someone and their destiny. What if you had the courage to share your story or to speak life to those around you? What if you became part of the solution to how God shakes the world of those around you? A key player in their story.

Why You?

Today, you are being called to wake up, to rise up and to go on a transformative journey.

What you hold in your heart and the abilities you possess are not small things. You have the power to shift the atmosphere around you. You are part of the solution to reviving the heart of medicine.

You have your own Personal Legend. It was written by the Author of the Universe, Jesus Christ. You have a great purpose to fulfill. Your life is meant to be a seed. Your story is in the process of being written. This is a pivotal time in history.

You must realize that you cannot afford to be asleep during this hour.

Your Moment and Your Choice

If you are in healthcare, you have the chance to take this amazing journey at a critical time in history. You have the chance to be on the frontlines of a new movement. If you are in any other field, you can use these keys to be the frontrunner of change in your industry. Regardless of your exact title, you must realize that this moment matters.

You are in a moment that requires decisive action. A Kairos moment. A time that was set apart. One where the Holy Spirit is moving, waiting to reveal the glory of Jesus Christ. He is calling you right now to co-labor with Him. At this moment, you and I have a choice to make. We must choose if we are to stay asleep and miss this movement or to step out in faith and become history-makers.

We have the chance to be part of His movement. Part of a group of people who are reviving the heart of medicine. Ones who have the courage to step out in a new way. Ones who will shift the atmosphere of healthcare for our colleagues, our patients and ourselves.

Similar to Santiago, the protagonist in the fictional story who was speaking to the wind and the sun, we are called to change the atmosphere in our field. In the lives of our coworkers and our patients.

As Christ followers, we know the only person who has the power to transform one completely, to give purpose and identity and to open one's eyes to their authority is Jesus

Christ. But here is the key. Christ lives in us. He lives in you and me. He is the key to reviving the heart of medicine. You must realize that you cannot lead others in this movement if you are not a good follower of Him.

You and Me

So, who is this book for? This book is for anyone who is interested in what the practice of medicine can and should be. It is for physicians, nurses, allied health professionals and any staff in clinical medicine who are seeking to bring healing to others. It is for family members of those in the healthcare field, as they are the support staff to those called to this mission. It is also for patients who want to be part of the frontlines as they witness how the atmosphere begins to shift in medicine. But it is especially for those who are burned out and looking to begin again. Those seeking meaning and hope in their life.

It is for you and me.

Your Journey

It is my goal in writing this book to wake up a generation that has been lulled to sleep by a broken healthcare system. One that has wandered far from its original roots.

It is my mission to help you discover the keys that unlock true healthcare. To help you learn what it looks like to bring the heart of the Father to your patients. To learn what it is to be led by the Holy Spirit in the field of medicine during these modern times. To show what practicing medicine can look like when done with the wisdom and guidance of the Great Physician, Jesus Christ and the Comforter, the Holy Spirit.

It is my mission to call forth an army of providers who are no longer willing to settle in the valley of the dry bones. To call forth leaders who will advocate for others at all costs.

I, and others in this book, are not special. Anyone with a heart for God and a spirit led by the Advocate can practice this way. We are only His seed. We have the chance to be used in the greater story that is revealing the glory of our Author.

You may be wondering if you have what it takes to transform spaces around you. The answer is a resounding yes. The only thing needed for your journey is a Heart to help others and a desire to walk with God. Eyes to see and Ears to hear. Senses that are finely tuned to your Maker. If you are breathing and if you are willing, God can move mountains through you.

Shifting Atmospheres

To be clear, I do not believe I can shift the wind or the sun on my own. I was told, though, that I could move mountains. I was told that there once was a man named Joshua who told the sun to stand still... and it did. I was told there was a God who clothed himself in humanity, who defied gravity and who walked on water and bid another to come... and he did. I was told of a God who became human who died for my sins and all others... and was resurrected on the third day. It was this same One who gave the commission,

"As you go, proclaim this message: 'The kingdom of heaven has come near.' Heal the sick, raise the dead, cleanse those who have

leprosy, drive out demons. Freely you have received; freely give."
Matthew 10:7-8, *NIV*

This commission stands today. To all who are willing to pursue it and the advancement of His kingdom.

So, if you are burned out from being part of a system that drains you of life and energy and are tired of carrying a burden that is too heavy for you to carry alone, this is for you. There is more.

We do not need more burned-out professionals. We need healthcare workers who burn for Him. We are called to be a light. We are called to light the flame in others. It is only when we are connected to our Source of light that we can begin to shift the atmosphere in our hospitals, clinics or even our homes.

We are not called to just practice medicine. We are called to revive the heart of medicine.

The Middle of a Miracle

"He is the one you praise; he is your God, who performed for you those great and awesome wonders you saw with your own eyes."
Deuteronomy 10:21 *NIV*

Do you have eyes to see? Have you seen God move? Do you have ears to hear? Have you heard God speak?

Jesus said,

"My sheep listen to my voice; I know them, and they follow me".
John 10:27 *NLT*

Do you know His voice? Are you familiar with its sound?

For those who have experienced God, their lives are forever changed. I'm not talking about head knowledge here.

I am talking about heart knowledge. I'm talking about when God becomes real to you.

We are told that He stands at the door and knocks, but we must do our part. We must be the ones to open the door. We must invite Him in. It is time for you to be handed the keys to open the door. To become familiar with His voice, His heart, and His mission in healthcare.

I am not starting you at the beginning of my journey. I am starting you in a moment where I first saw God move in radical ways. A time when I witnessed my first miracle in healthcare. I am starting you in a moment where I witnessed God become real in the life of my patient. Where I first saw God truly shift the atmosphere in a hospital room.

Why am I starting you here? Because you need to know where you are journeying. You need to know there is amazing breakthrough if you have the courage to move forward in pursuing God's heart in medicine.

You must know there is a treasure to be found. You must desire to learn the keys to help you on your own journey.

You may be wondering, what happened before I saw God move in radical ways? It is simple. I was praying. Soaking in time with Him. Enjoying who He is. Experiencing the essence of prayer. Talking with God. Hearing what is on His heart. Giving Him my praises, worries, cares, and concerns. It is in prayer that your journey starts. It is in prayer that my ears were opened.

I must clarify a few things first though regarding prayer. There is praying in the Spirit, praying in your native language, and there are times when we just spend time with our Friend, soaking in His presence. It was the last one that got me that night. It happened the night before I really saw

God move in the life of my patient. I still remember the night that this first happened, when I learned what it meant to be silent.

Do you know those special times when you enjoy the silence and company of those closest to you? You don't have to exchange any words. You just soak in the atmosphere. There is peace and comfort just being in each other's presence.

The same is true with the Lord. It is in times of silence, in just spending time with your closest friend, the Holy Spirit, when He will speak to you in the most radical way.

That night, we were in our living room, and my husband and I were just listening to worship music and relaxing, soaking in His presence. Worshipping Him in our hearts and enjoying the peaceful atmosphere. It came out of nowhere. It was a boy's name that popped into my mind, seemingly out of nowhere. It came again. I heard it repeated twice.

Hmm. That was odd. I was not thinking of anything along those lines, and yet, the name appeared clearly and was spoken in my heart two times. It was an uncommon name. Not the name of anyone that I knew.

I was perplexed. I spoke to my husband about it. As is common, I discussed it with him and asked if he knew of anyone with that name or if he knew of a reason I would hear that name so clearly, not once, but twice. He was just as confused as I was. So, I sat with it and realized I would know what it meant when the time was right.

That's the thing about God's words. Sometimes the word He gives is a right now word, but sometimes, it is a word for the future. Either way, He will reveal to you and open your eyes to the meaning of the word in His time. Well, that was the night before Thanksgiving.

As I woke up on Thanksgiving morning, I quickly showered and prepared for my shift in the Emergency Department. I prayed that God would reveal to me the meaning of the name and why I heard it. I heard nothing. As the morning went on, I grew comfortable with not knowing. More than that, I was actually looking forward to my time in the Emergency Department.

Typically, the morning of a holiday in an Emergency Department is quite slow. Most people are enjoying their time with family and friends. It is not until later in the day that the crazy happens. It is not until late in the shift when things really pick up. That is the pace on a normal holiday. Yet, I found out quickly that today was not a normal day.

As I badged in at 6 am and walked through those double doors, something was different. It was not a scene that I was expecting to see. I walked by a room and noticed there were three physicians in the room. It was very crowded. Not only was it crowded, but there was also a lot of activity.

Hmm, that's odd, I thought. Why was there an anesthesiologist, a surgeon and the night emergency medicine physician at the bedside of a patient? That scene is more typical in a larger hospital. One that typically sees a lot of trauma patients. But in our small Emergency Department, that is not a common sight. Now, I was really intrigued.

I waited for the doctor to come and give me sign-out. She began to fill me in on the patients who she was handing off to me. She went quickly through the list so she could focus on the one in that crowded room. The little boy who was now on a ventilator.

I asked her why the boy was so sick. She went on to tell me how things unfolded over the night. She said the boy had been brought in by family for shortness of breath. She then said that within a 2-hour period, she saw the boy rapidly progress into full respiratory failure. She had done all the typical non-invasive support such as nebulizer treatments, supplemental oxygen through a nasal cannula, steroids, etc. Yet, nothing helped.

Over time, she realized the boy was getting progressively more tired. His body was unable to sustain the effort that was required to keep the breath in his lungs. So, she did what any good Emergency Medicine physician would do. She sedated him, intubated him and placed him on a ventilator.

This is where things turned for the worse. She had done everything right, but the boy just got sicker. She had gotten the post-intubation x-ray and confirmed the tube in his trachea was in the right place, but still, the boy was not clinically improving. His oxygen levels continued to drop, even with maxed-out settings on the ventilator. Things should be shifting in the right direction by now but they were not.

One of the boy's lungs appeared very white or opaque on the chest x-ray. There was a mucous plug, a block in the airway, that was preventing oxygen from fully penetrating his lungs. This is when she called in the anesthesiologist and a surgeon. She started with the surgeon. She asked him to do a bronchoscope in an attempt to clear the debris. Here was the catch.

We are not a pediatric or critical care hospital. We were working in a tiny rural hospital that did not have all the supplies we needed. This boy was very young. There was no scope small enough to suction the mucous from his distal airways.

The surgeon looked defeated. What was he supposed to do? His skills were useless at this point. That left the anesthesiologist. He was trying different settings on the ventilator. Addressing volume, rate, and pressure settings. Still no changes.

It was at this point that I had come on shift. I did not know who this boy was, but I was going to assume his care, so I had better get to know him. I walked into the room and just stood there. I watched as the three other physicians in the room were standing there, trying to decide the next steps. Waiting for a transfer to a children's hospital that was delayed.

I forgot to mention that it was terrible weather this morning. It was well into fall, and there was thick fog and snow, which was common in our region. The pediatric transfer team had not been given the signal that they could safely fly, so the waiting game began.

In the natural, it seemed like all hope was lost. Looking at the scientific facts, this boy was not going to survive this, whatever *"this"* was. The atmosphere was bleak.

The boy's oxygen levels were staying at 86% on the monitor. This is not sufficient to oxygenate his vital organs and tissues for a sustained period of time. The oxygen level was not budging. It's like the monitor was taunting us.

So, I did the next thing I thought of. I laid my hands on the boy's feet. I prayed for wisdom. I prayed for an answer. I prayed for anything, God. I heard *"N-acetylcysteine"* pop into my mind. Hmm. Okay, let's go with it. I knew this medication thinned secretions, and I knew this boy had a mucous plug. It couldn't hurt. It could only help.

So, I asked the anesthesiologist if they had tried N-acetylcysteine. They hadn't. He thought it was a great idea. We had the respiratory therapist begin to nebulize this for the patient. We watched. All of us waiting to see the 86% increase to at least 92%. We kept waiting.

Yet, nothing happened.

We waited another 15 minutes. No change whatsoever. Okay, the next thing that came to mind was proning. Had this boy been turned onto his stomach to improve the ventilation of his lungs, or had we placed the boy on his side with his bad lung higher towards the ceiling? Had we tried this? No, this had not been done.

Our team grew hopeful once again. We worked together, carefully trying to keep all tubing in place and not getting too tangled up when we flipped the boy over. We stood there. We waited. Come on! We need the oxygen saturation to budge. We needed it to get to at least 92%. We collectively seemed to hold our own breath, waiting.

Again, nothing happened.

We waited another 15 minutes. Yet, again, no change. Now, I was beginning to really worry for this boy. I did not know who he was or who he belonged to, but my heart was breaking for him. The team was discouraged.

I heard the surgeon now say he had nothing more he could add, so he was going to begin his rounds and help other patients. He opened the door and left. Next was the anesthesiologist. He said he had done everything he could think of to do. He was out of solutions, so he was the next to leave.

This left the other Emergency physician and myself. Two women in the room. One a non-believer and one a believer. I heard it then. Clearly. I sensed it so strongly in my spirit. *"This one is going to require prayer."* It was quiet but it was very strong. An urgent request to partner with God on this case. A sense of fear immediately washed over me.

Thoughts began to tumble through my mind, *"Really, God? Am I supposed to pray over this boy for his healing? How is this going to work? I mean, I know how to pray, but this other physician doesn't even believe in God, and I don't know what this family's thoughts are on this."* The thoughts were increasing in pace. God wasn't impressed. My arguments did not seem to matter. I heard the same instruction. *"Pray."*

So, I did what I could think of next. It was not courageous. It was not earth shattering. I decided to distract the other doctor. I sent her out of the room and told her to go do charts. I told her I would stay with the boy.

She seemed reluctant to leave. I had not given her any reason or any game plan. She must have sensed I had made up my mind and wasn't going to budge. So, she was the next to slide open the door and walk out of the room.

I took a deep breath in and walked over to the curtains. I quickly closed the curtains. I told you, I didn't claim to be brave. I then looked at the father and the grandfather. They were the only family members in the room. I spoke the next thing that came to me. *"How are you doing?"*

The words tumbled out of their mouth in unison, *"I'm scared"*. I knew that was my cue. My open door.

That's the thing about caring for our patients. If you have ears to hear, you will hear when your door creaks opens.

You must continually be on the lookout for these open window and door *"opportunities."*

I took my open door and ran. I asked them if they would be okay praying with me over the boy. Immediately, I sensed relief in their voices. Without hesitation, they both said, *"yes"*. I asked them next to come up to the bed. To get out of their seats and lay hands on the boy. To watch the tubing, but to find any area where they could lay their hands and begin to intercede on this boy's behalf.

It was then that I realized. I had been with this boy for 2 hours. I had been so focused on his vital signs and on the plan to get him better, but I had missed his name. How could I pray for him and not know his name?

So, as I was starting the prayer, I shifted his patient's wristband enough to learn his name. There it was. In black and white. The boy's name I had heard the night prior when I was spending time with the Holy Spirit. The same name I had heard when I was taking time to hear what was on God's heart.

I was rattled.

I took a deep breath in and began the prayer. It was not an eloquent prayer. I believe I fumbled over my words a bit. I was nervous. Yet, even in my brokenness, the atmosphere began to shift in the room. It was subtle at first but it kept growing stronger. I could physically feel His presence. Heaven was invading Earth at that very moment. It felt almost like a stirring of wind, something that was very subtle, but it was a flood of peace that filled that room.

I finished the prayer in Jesus' name. There wasn't a dry eye as I walked out of the room. I was now the final physician to close the door. As I did, I patted the grandpa's hand and told him, *"Your boy is in good hands now".*

I slid the door closed and went back to the provider's office. I sat at my desk. Drained. The monitor glared overhead. I was quite visibly shaken after this experience, but I needed to be able to focus on the other patients in my care. It had been two hours since arriving on shift. Two hours of seeing his vitals not change. Stubborn and hovering at 86%.

Hope Rising

It was 5 minutes later that I looked up. I could not believe my eyes. I was watching the monitor go up in real time.

87%

88%

89%

Pause

90%

91%

92%

And it held....

It stayed at 92%!!!

It was not a perfect oxygen saturation level but it became the new set point for the boy. I could not believe my eyes. Did this just happen? I mean, I know we are to believe in miracles, but when you are in the middle of one, you often cannot believe what you are seeing.

It reminded me of the story in Acts 12 when Peter showed up at Mary's house, and the servant girl was so excited that she left Peter out in the cold. She left the miracle they had been praying for out in the elements. She could not believe that their prayers had worked, and that Peter had been released from the prison.

That is the thing when you begin to believe in miracles, and you begin to ask Heaven to invade Earth. There are times when you will be astonished to see the hand of God move in your situation.

Well, it was at that moment that I witnessed and registered this miracle that we got the phone call. The fog had broken. The transfer team had been cleared to fly. They were leaving now and would be here in about an hour. Specialized care for this boy was on the way. God had broken through the enemy's plans for this boy. He was sending relief.

As that phone call was ending, the other physician burst into the provider's office. She had been doing charts but then had walked by the nurses' station and saw the monitor. She saw the new set point. She saw that the boy was now safe.

She burst into the provider office and said directly, *"What did you do in there? Why were the curtains closed?"* I told her the first thing that came to mind. I told her the truth, *"I prayed over the boy with his family."* The next thing that popped out of my mouth was, *"Where science and medicine failed, God stepped in"*.

She was silent. She was now the one processing the miracle. You could tell she didn't know what to believe. Her mind was so filled and set on scientific facts, yet her reality was just shaken by the movement of God. Now, she had to decide what her next move would be. Would she open the door for Him in her own heart?

She had seen with her own eyes that the boy had been

critically ill, not changing for hours. She had been the one to intubate him. She had been the one to keep seeing failure and dead ends with treatment. And then, in a moment, after a time in prayer, he was now in a safe zone. He was now able to more adequately oxygenate his tissues. She could not deny the truth.

The only thing in between the state of our patient's critical condition and now his improved condition and vitals on the monitor was prayer. The unbeliever had just witnessed the power of God in medicine. Looking back on this day, I still do not know how this moment truly impacted that clinician. I hope that this moment planted a seed. I hope that a physical healing of a boy was not the only healing that occurred that day. Time will tell.

To our excitement and relief though, the boy's vitals remained steady until the critical transport team arrived. He remained steady during the flight and was safely transported to the other hospital. He had arrived under the care of physicians who had more specialized equipment and more trained teams than us.

He may have left our little hospital, but he did not go alone. The Lord went with him. The boy was being held and protected by the Great Physician. He was truly in the best of hands. That was only the beginning though...

I will tell you more about this boy's discharge in a bit. My shift was far from over. My adrenaline was now tapped. I felt exhausted from such a stressful period, followed by a miraculous breakthrough, and my body didn't know what to expect next. It was then that I heard our EMS phone ring. They were again calling in on the radio. They were bringing in a pediatric trauma patient who had been injured on an ATV.

Oh, man. My heart sank. This was supposed to be an easy shift! Really?! Another pediatric critical patient?! I barely just got the other one out of here! I pleaded silently that this one would go much smoother.

It was only about 20 minutes later that EMS was bringing the gurney through the large ambulance bay door. The boy was a similar age to the other one I had sent out. This boy was screaming in pain and was holding his deformed leg.

Our team moved into the trauma bay and began the primary survey. Airway - intact. He was definitely screaming. Breathing - symmetric chest rise noted. Auscultation of the lungs revealed bilateral breath sounds. Mentation - I was at the head of the bed when I asked the boy his name. I asked him if he could repeat it to me.

I remember that moment so clearly to this day. The boy stopped screaming for a moment. Just long enough to focus and answer the question he had been asked. He looked straight up at me with his bright blue eyes, tears filling them, and he spoke his name. It was the same name from the night prior. The same name as the boy I had just shipped out to the other hospital. Gasp.

Think Twice

Now, it was my turn to check my breath. I couldn't believe what I had just heard. Two boys with the same name, on the same shift, that I had been given a heads up on the night prior.

It finally clicked that God had revealed ahead of time that He was going to be sending me two boys during my shift. Two boys who had an important role to play. These were obviously extra special patients. Not that all patients are not special to God, but there was something different about these boys that the Holy Spirit decided to give an advanced warning about.

Cases that would require me to be extra focused. Patients where I must trust His wisdom over my head knowledge. Ones that needed me to be an advocate when they could not advocate for themselves.

Thankfully, this boy had less serious injuries than the first and was in less critical condition than the boy on the ventilator. He had some broken bones that were going to require us to ship him to the same children's hospital as the other boy, but he was going to be fine.

As I was getting ready to splint him, I took a moment to speak identity into the boy. I had looked up the name that I had been given the night before. I had realized that if God was taking the time to speak a name to me, I should at least know what it means. So, as the tech was wrapping up his leg, I asked the boy a question. *"Do you know what your name means?"*

He looked up at me again with his bright blue eyes and said *"no"*. He then looked at his parents with curiosity and asked them. They also did not know.

I told him one of the meanings of his name is *"Warrior"*. I told him, *"You are a warrior!"* I didn't stop there, though. I wanted to make sure that his identity soaked into who he was. I wanted him to remember this day not for the bad accident but for the good he learned about himself. A day that he will remember during stressful times ahead. I told him, *"You are brave and courageous, and you have amazing things ahead of you!"*

The boy took a deep breath in. You could tell he was in pain getting the splint on. He breathed in one more time and shouted, *"Did you hear that?! I am a warrior!!!"*. The whole room erupted in laughter, including his parents.

That's the thing with words and speaking identity over your patients. It costs you nothing, yet it is priceless. Others gain so much from words that are a blessing. The power of the tongue is unsurpassed when used to speak life over others in your path. The right words spoken over someone have the power to shift their destiny. The right words that you speak over yourself can shape who you are and what you will become. There is a reason we are to guard not only our hearts but also our words.

If you take a moment to think about the enemy's current strategy, in this day and age, it is a war that is waged on identity. The enemy wants there to be confusion and discord with one's identity. You do not have to fall for the lies of the enemy. Those who come across your path can be lifted up by the Truth. Darkness is broken by light.

We have the power of life and death in our tongues. Each day, we must make a choice. Will we speak life, or will we speak death? Will we repeat the enemy's lies over us, or will we speak God's truth?

God has given you the authority to speak to your mountains. He is the one who will do the hard work. He is just looking for those brave enough to take Him at His word and speak to those mountains.

Overruled

Well, both warriors got shipped off that day. Boys with different wounds but warriors that God has an amazing mission for. Ones that God decided to pull back the spiritual realm's veil for, bringing a piece of heaven into that small emergency department that day. I am certain of this.

A couple of weeks later, I got the reports back from the other hospital. My patient on the ventilator should have died multiple times during the hospitalization. He defied the odds, though. God broke through and showed out. He kept him safe against all the circumstances that said otherwise. The boy made it through the whole hospitalization. He was discharged in stable condition.

God said overruled. He overruled the plans of the enemy for both of those boys that day. It was a Thanksgiving for which God showed me just how many things there were to be thankful for.

The Power of Prayer

That is the thing with prayer. You never know what secrets you will learn or what words of knowledge you will be given. You never know if your prayer is going to mean the difference between life and death for someone. You never know when God will call you to intercede on another's behalf.

Why do you pray? Why do you seek to know the Holy Spirit intimately? Why do we need to revive the heart of medicine?

So that you can truly become a friend of God. When you listen and actually hear, you can go after the things that are on His heart. You can walk daily being led by His Spirit. You can be obedient when He tells you to move. You can stop when He tells you to stop.

Even if it costs you greatly, you must step forward in faith. You never know just what miracles He has in mind. What moves He wants you to do. You never fully know the ways that He wants to move through you to reach others. You never know how your words will be used to shift someone's personal atmosphere.

What about you? Are you willing to spend time with God in prayer? Are you willing to hear His secrets? Are you willing to become a friend of the Holy Spirit? Are you willing to be His advocate? To contend for the breakthrough that your patients so desperately need?

That is the Personal Legend. That is the answer to shifting the atmosphere of healthcare. The secret to reviving the heart of medicine. But it is only just the beginning. You have seen what you are seeking. Now you need the keys.

Before you learn of these, you must take a few moments to see where healthcare is at this current moment. You must see where the starting point is so that you know how necessary this journey truly is. You must open your eyes and see clearly why the heart of medicine must be revived. You must open your heart and know who the true Healer really is.

..."If you will listen carefully to the voice of the LORD your God and do what is right in his sight, obeying his commands and keeping all his decrees, then I will not make you suffer any of the diseases I sent on the Egyptians; for I am the LORD who heals you."
Exodus 15:26 *NLT*

Rattled

"Then the Lord God formed the man of dust from the ground and breathed into his nostrils the breath of life, and the man became a living creature."
Genesis 2:7 *ESV*

Right now, we have an army of dead healthcare workers. That may sound harsh. I meant it to. I can say this. I was once one of them. These healthcare workers have been mortally wounded by the system and by the enemy. They are the ones whose hearts need to be spiritually revived.

That's why I didn't start you out with this truth in the first chapter. You would have immediately closed the book. I needed to start you out with hope, and there is hope. There is a great hope. There is a way out of our current situation in healthcare. However, you must accurately see the current situation if you are going to make it to the other side.

You are smart. You already understand that you can't treat what you have not correctly diagnosed. You learned in the first chapter what it is like to practice medicine when you are "*alive*." When your heart is revived and beating for Him. When you have been awakened by the Holy Spirit and are seeking after hearing His voice.

But, before I learned the things we will be speaking of more in this book, I was asleep. My heart was dry and cracked. My main goal was just trying to make it through each day. Each shift, I would show up and watch the little life I had get sucked out of me. I was going through the motions. Afraid to step out or speak up as that would call unwanted attention to myself. Burned out. Frustrated with the daily grind. Frustrated with the lack of seeing real change in patients and the emptiness in my colleagues.

These healthcare workers are great people! Many have good hearts. They are in a noble profession. I call many of them my friends. What you and I are experiencing is real. We are not wrong for feeling this way. The sad part, though, is that many blame themselves for these feelings. Many don't allow themselves to feel what they are rightfully allowed to feel.

They would never say this, but they sense they are missing something. Those who are honest and in touch with themselves feel weak because they feel this way. This could not be further from the truth. They have just been misled. They have been lulled to sleep. They have gone into a protective response and hardened themselves and their hearts against a broken system.

They haven't had anyone tell them the truth. They have

been blinded to the truth that the heart of medicine has grown dry and bitter. It is a barren landscape. Until now.

What many don't realize is that the true issue behind this is the fact that healthcare is dead. Not in the physical sense, but in the spiritual. Healthcare needs a remedy, and it needs it now. It needs its atmosphere to be shifted. It needs its heart to be revived.

Workers know something is wrong with healthcare, but they were taught over the past few years that they couldn't speak up. That would be too difficult. Too risky. They learned that it was safer for them to be part of a majority. To not question. To just show up and be a good soldier. They believed it was someone else's battle to fight.

They didn't have the energy to break out of the status quo. Many thought they didn't need to. They accepted what was put on the plate in front of them, and they were acquiescent when handing it out. They are good people caught up in a broken system.

Losing the War

It started insidiously at first. So subtle that many didn't even realize the slow fade. The oxygen was slowly being sucked out of the room. They were slowly losing their breath. Little gasps here and there. The breath that once sustained them escaped their lungs.

It was gradual, but it continued to slip away. Little by little. One gasp at a time. What started slowly, though, gained momentum, much like any revolution. Before they knew it, they had joined the valley of the dry bones. An army that had fallen asleep while on guard. Ones that had experienced a mortal blow that they could not wake from... on their own.

Was it healthcare that Ezekial spoke about all those years ago? Was it this army that he was shown? I think so. It's at least one of the armies. It seems like many others have fallen asleep as well. Listen to the words Ezekial spoke of and you decide.

"I felt the power of the Lord on me, and he brought me out by the Spirit of the Lord and put me down in the middle of a valley. It was full of bones. He led me around among the bones, and I saw that there were many bones in the valley and that they were very dry. Then he asked me, "Human, can these bones live?"

I answered, "Lord God, only you know."

He said to me, "Prophesy to these bones and say to them, 'Dry bones, hear the word of the Lord. This is what the Lord God says to the bones: I will cause breath to enter you so you will come to life. I will put muscles on you and flesh on you and cover you with skin. Then I will put breath in you so you will come to life. Then you will know that I am the Lord."

So, I prophesied as I was commanded. While I prophesied, there was a noise and a rattling. The bones came together, bone to bone. I looked and saw muscles come on the bones, and flesh grew, and skin covered the bones. But there was no breath in them.

Then he said to me, "Prophesy to the wind. Prophesy, human, and say to the wind, 'This is what the Lord God says: Wind, come from the four winds, and breathe on these people who were killed so they can come back to life.'"

So, I prophesied as the Lord commanded me. And the breath

came into them, and they came to life and stood on their feet, a very large army.
Ezekial 37: 1-10 (*New Century Version*)

The Division of Healthcare

What was it that caused the mortal blow? What was it that sent this army into a downward spiral? It was a long, weary battle over several years. One focused on financial gain and lacking, at times, in integrity. It was finished off with the arrows from the most recent Pandemic. Wounds that were caused by the enemy of all our souls. A battle that was openly played out in the healthcare arena.

Before you decide to shut your eyes and avoid something that you would like to leave alone, take a moment to be open-minded and think. A moment that may shift the rest of your life. Think back. What dominated the atmosphere in homes in America during the Pandemic? What dominated the atmosphere of healthcare across the globe?

It was fear and division. Plain and simple.

Anyone who was a first responder or who practiced in the realm of patient care during this period of time has a multitude of stories about what it was like to practice medicine during the Pandemic. Anyone who was a patient during the Pandemic (i.e. all of us) has many stories of what it was like to be a patient or to have a family member or friend as a patient during that time period.

I can tell you with confidence that the providers and the patients alike will not speak of peace when describing this era. They will not speak of reconciliation. They will not speak fondly of this period. No. Most definitely, they will not.

They will come forward, many with tears in their eyes. Tears that only begin to express the pain they went through. They will speak of losing friendships. Losing loved ones. Feeling shame. Anger. Isolation. Helplessness.

They will speak of an atmosphere that changed how they looked at the world around them. How they lost trust in medicine. How they lost trust in their friendships, trust in their families, trust in their leaders. An atmosphere that literally sucked the life out of all of us.

The Aftershocks

Most providers and patients to this day are still experiencing the aftershocks of the shakings that permeated the COVID Pandemic. An atmosphere that shifted modern medicine and the world attached to it.

Although I can only speak from my experience in the American healthcare system as an Emergency Medicine physician during this time, I can tell you that the atmosphere of healthcare shifted when COVID reached our shores. Fear and dread were the first two horsemen to arrive in this health apocalypse. These arrived from a long distance and taunted patients and healthcare providers alike.

Division was the third horseman to arrive, followed by anger and isolation. Division of how best to treat patients and how best to protect staff. Division of which side of the fence you fell on. Were you going to make *the choice* or not?

Phrases that were repeated in people's daily lives, such as

"How dare you!" if you chose not to follow the yellow brick road. "Are you not loving?" and *"How could you be thinking the way you are thinking?"*. These were the catchphrases of the time.

These sound like the lies of the enemy. Words that cause harm, not healing. Words that are filled with partial truths yet lead one down the path of destruction. These were not the words of a healthcare provider whose job is to bring health and promote healing.

Yet, you already know this. You guessed it. You heard it. How can I say this so confidently? Because I know that you already lived it. We both did. You may not be aware of it, but you experienced cancel culture to the extreme. You lived through a culture that kills.

An environment where family members accused other family members. Doctors accused other doctors, and nurses turned on their colleagues. And administration? Well, they retreated to their boardrooms as they did not fully know what to do. They tried to legislate "safety" while promoting division and isolation.

Patients? They were left trying to find the truth. Trying to find answers. Trying not to be shamed while seeking help.

Can you feel the atmosphere? It is palpable. It is dark. The air was being sucked out of our lungs. One hurt at a time. One cruel word at a time.

What do you sense when you read all of this? I imagine you are remembering what you went through during these past few years. Let me take a moment to stop and say I am truly sorry for the hurt you and I experienced. I am sorry for those who hurt you and those you lost. I am sorry you felt vulnerable and unprotected.

Know that you are worthy. You are loved beyond measure. There is hope.

Bandaging the Wounds

Some may want to stop reading here, and that would be unfortunate. You must recognize these wounds if you are going to grow in a manner you never thought possible. You must open your eyes if you are going to be part of the solution to reviving medicine.

What do you notice about the first descriptions above? Do you feel at peace reading them? Or did you hear the shouting voice of the accuser? Were you becoming uncomfortable? That's okay. Those are legitimate feelings. You can't deal with something you won't face. You must lance the abscess if it's going to heal. You cannot resuscitate what you will not touch.

The atmosphere of medicine was truly a messy landscape during COVID. It's still messy now. That's why we need those with the courage to confront it head-on. We must shift the atmosphere of medicine. We must revive that which is currently dead.

It is no longer an option. We must not settle for the last several years. We must realize that physical "heart attacks" are not as detrimental as spiritual "heart attacks". As a medical community, we accept the fact that scar tissue forms when one has a myocardial infarction, aka heart attack, and this causes irreversible damage to one's heart. This damage can prevent the heart from beating correctly and functioning as effectively as it should. If the heart attack affects too much of the heart, then the person will not survive the event.

Timing and correct treatment matter. A Band-Aid or an essential oil is not going to cut it when one is having a physical heart attack. Spiritually, our hearts can experience the same thing. When there are too many hurts that are not quickly dealt with, damage occurs. When spiritual roots are left in place, they can corrupt and rot one's whole being. Scar tissue forms and the enemy continues to work.

We must effectively address these roots if we are to be healed and whole. Furthermore, we need to realize that we cannot truly heal our patients if we have not dealt with the damage in our own hearts. We have to have hearts that are effectively beating if we are to fulfill the calling on our lives. We must wake up and realize that healing always begins from the inside out. An aspirin is not going to cut it this time.

Remembering our First Love

We must truly come back to life again. To have our dry hearts become filled with the blood of Life again. Hearts that beat for others. Hearts that beat with the love of the Father.

We must remember the Hippocratic Oath that we once spoke. We must remember our once shared goal of protecting patients and our fellow man, no matter the cost. We must remember what it means to be an advocate.

We were never meant to exchange accusations of selfishness if one chose a different path than us. No! That is not the atmosphere of medicine we will accept. That is the voice and actions of the accuser of our soul.

We were never meant to overhear or have conversations in halls that certain patients *"deserved this"* and hear other conversations where providers or staff were being openly mocked. How can such toxicity exist in a healing environment? How can you heal others when you are spewing such poison?

Take a look in the mirror. Do you recognize yourself? Are you who you want to be? It's time to open your eyes. Not in judgment but in grace. We must assess the damage and make the necessary adjustments. Survey the damage and come up with a plan. There is a better way.

This is not why we went into a field to bind up the broken. We were never meant to be the ones doing the breaking. We are called higher than that. You are called higher than that.

Grace in the Storm

The atmosphere during the Pandemic was poisoned with pride, anger and unforgiveness. It was darkened further with the fear of uncertainty. It was not only healthcare workers who were suffocated by this toxic environment. It was the patients.

Patients who lost hope in their previously trusted providers. Patients who lost hope that they would be treated fairly when they sought care. Patients who lost trust that others would not judge or demean them for their choices during the pandemic.

An atmosphere that was thick like a heavy wet blanket. Pressing one down and causing exhaustion. Causing a slow fade.

Not all was lost, though, in this tempestuous atmosphere. God was still there. God's love was ever present. There were glimmers of hope. Glimmers of love, if you were brave enough to listen and look.

There were moments of courage and standing together. There were first responders and those who risked their lives to save others. Some won the battle, and some lost it, making the ultimate sacrifice. These we are forever grateful to. These heroes were examples of pure love, mercy, and grace in the midst of the storm.

Why am I painting this picture? Why am I reminding you of a period that most of us would choose to forget? Because you need to recognize that there is a bigger picture at play. You need to realize what put you and me to sleep. You must understand what drained the life out of our friends and loved ones.

The enemy was using division, anger, unforgiveness and isolation in healthcare to literally suck the life out of patients and healthcare providers alike.

Look Again

It was not just a virus that we were battling with. We were not just wrestling with flesh and blood but with principalities. Principalities that shifted the atmosphere of medicine. A virus that infected the heart of medicine.

And it was not only medicine that was left tarnished. Principalities also sought to break down personal, corporate, financial, and governmental walls. These walls are still damaged today. But God didn't let the enemy have the last say. He never does.

God used what the enemy meant to harm us with and turned it around for our good. He began to wake people up.

He began revealing what was truly at play and what was at stake. He began to reveal the true atmosphere of medicine and what it could become if we woke up. He began to reveal that the heart of medicine must be revived by His character and His love.

Speak Life

He began speaking life into the army. Into our dry bones. Into those with eyes to see and ears to hear.

It happened slowly at first, but they began to wake up and recognize the poisonous environment they were surrounded by. An atmosphere polluted with division, fear, uncertainty, anger and unforgiveness. An atmosphere that was too toxic to survive in. One sickened with pride. One that inflicted massive wounds on the providers and patients alike.

You may be wondering what the good part of all of this is. Don't give up, it is here.

Wake up and Push Back

We do not have to settle here in this environment. We do not have to accept the current atmosphere of medicine. You do not have to settle in the valley of the dry bones. If you are still reading this book, then I am sure you realize there is a remedy. You are seeking it. That's an amazing thing!

We were given a promise that if we seek Him, we will find Him. You can claim this promise today. You must realize that God always brings good out of ALL things and redeems ALL things for those who love Him. Know that He is going after redeeming not only this period of time but redeeming the field of medicine. Shifting the atmosphere in which His healers practice.

He is not sitting idly by and doing nothing. No. He is entreating us to partner with Him to shift the tide. To push back the darkness that is pervasive right now in medicine. He is asking those who are courageous enough to seek Him for answers to worldly issues. To ask Heaven to invade the Earth.

He wants to give heavenly instruction and knowledge to the simple so that we will be strong in Him. He wants us to reflect His character of mercy and grace. To reflect His self-less love for His people.

He is calling a group of providers who are willing to step out, risk everything, and consecrate themselves to shift the atmosphere of medicine. To revive the heart of medicine.

He is asking us to push back the principalities and stand in the gap for our patients. To receive healing ourselves for the hurts inflicted from this period of time so that we can be the ones to bring reconciliation to others.

The atmosphere of medicine must shift from that of division to one of reconciliation. The heart of medicine must be turned from a dry, barren landscape into a heart that beats for Him again.

You must wake up. You are the solution. You have a powerful purpose. You are an advocate. It is your job to co-labor with God in resuscitating the heart of medicine.

No more should you be willing to sit here idle. To look at your job as just another thing on your to-do list. There is great work ahead of you and me, and it's going to require an army of His powerful believers to bring it to life again. It's going to take both you and me to change the world around us. It is going to take fresh insight and revelation to begin again.

He is the key to reviving the heart of medicine.

Do you hear it? Do you sense it? Can you hear the rattle? I sure can. I hear the sound of many feet walking out of a valley of dry bones back into the land of the living.

ENCOUNTER

"You will seek me and find me when you seek me with all your heart."
Jeremiah 29:13 *NIV*

Have you ever heard something that stopped you in your tracks? Something that sank an anchor into you quicker than you realized.

Well, that happened to me recently at a leadership conference. I was sitting there enjoying the lecture when I heard the words, *"To be a good leader, you must first be a good follower. A follower of Christ, that is."*

You could have heard a feather land in the auditorium with how quiet the room got after those words were spoken. A very simple statement, but one that was absolutely profound. One that caught everyone's attention. A basic concept that I inherently knew but one I hadn't personally heard uttered before.

While that is absolutely true for leadership, I believe it is much broader than that. The more I have lived, the more I have realized that anyone worth following must first be a true follower of Christ. Don't throw up your hands in defense. This is not about religion. It is about relationship.

Relationship with the heart of the Father. One that is not legalistic but a relationship that is all consuming. One where knowledge is transformed into revelation. One that has the power to transform every area of your life.

There is no lukewarm when it comes to God. At least no lukewarm when it comes to being usable by Him. There is no sitting on the sidelines and just hoping to bide our time waiting for Heaven to come. No! We are called to bring His kingdom to others. We are called to be the change that we want to see. We are called to reflect the heart of the Father. To be led by the Holy Spirit, the Spirit of wisdom. By our actions and not just words, we are called to lead others to His son, Jesus Christ.

It took me several years of being a *"Christian"* to get this concept. Several years sitting on the pews and half-heartedly singing *"His Kingdom Come"* before I even knew what that meant.

My journey to being on fire for God included a wilderness season. A season of hitting the lowest of lows and completely going off course for a few years. The short story is that it was a prodigal season for me.

Thank God, He included the story of the Prodigal Son in the Bible and that He uses people who are not qualified. Thank God that in my weakness, I am made stronger. Even more so, thank God He didn't leave me in my mess. He reached down and pulled me from the deep waters.

God does not leave us alone in the valleys where we

failed. God calls us up higher. He calls us into an encounter with Him. He calls us to a much higher place. A place where He is seated on the throne.

So, the first key on your journey is all about going from head knowledge of God to heart knowledge. It is a necessary step that takes place when you see the God of Abraham, Isaac, and Jacob come to life. When you see Him move for the first time. When you hear as He speaks directly to you.

It is when you experience the move of God in your life in such a way that you begin to experience who He truly is. You begin to see that He is worthy to be followed. That He is always with you, and He is for you.

Life with God is anything but boring. He often restores our vision and focus on Him in the most unusual of ways.

Dream Life

Me, I still remember being shaken the first time that God spoke to me. The first time I truly knew that He moved on my behalf. It was in a dream where the Holy Spirit first spoke to me. He met me in one of my darkest moments. When my atmosphere was very bleak.

It was in a period of time when I had just heard a *"knock, knock"* at my door. When I opened it, the man standing there looked awkward. I could sense the pity. It was then that I learned what it meant to be served divorce papers.

I was nearing the end of my first year of medical school when I heard that knock. The day when I clearly remember my world came crashing down. Yes. To put it lightly, it was not a pleasant time.

As a medical student, I was used to seeing a lot of papers.

But these were papers I never thought I would see. Papers that I had grown up knowing were not for me.

You see, I had married my high school sweetheart. I had grown up in the church. I had married someone who I thought I would be with forever. I had a beautiful wedding, wore a beautiful satin and lace dress and was sure that I was on my way to my happily ever after. Everything seemed great, until it wasn't.

I won't go over the details, but I will say that I was crushed. I could not think straight. I went from a *"we"* to a *"me"* in a short period of time, and my head was left spinning. It was at the end of my first year of medical school that this crushing occurred. A time shortly prior to finals.

That's one of the most amazing things about God. He often encounters us most strongly in our darkest moments. In times when we believe there's no way, things can turn around for good.

Well, I was in southern California at the time, and there was no amount of sunshine that could snap me out of the fog I seemed to be suffocated by. The atmosphere would just not let up. During this period of time, my brain was not functioning. And as a medical student, you really need your brain to function.

Well, finals were rapidly approaching. I was struggling to show up to classes and to absorb the fire hose of information that was being given to me as a medical student. I was limping by.

That was, except for one class. The biggest class of the first year. This class was called PDx – Patient Diagnosis. And it was a beast. To be honest, I was less than limping by in this class. I was like a slug that had been thrown against a wall, and I was slowly following the path of gravity.

Well, to pass the first year, I had to pass this class. The teacher who taught this class was tough. His curriculum was not as sweet as the Dr. Pepper he loved to drink every day while he was up on the podium. He was determined to pull everything out of each student that he could. He was relentless. So was his course.

As the day of the final exam approached, the more nervous I got. I was glumly staring at the pages of the massive study guide but could not seem to retain any of the information swirling around in my head. I tried and kept trying, but it felt useless. Have you ever felt that way? Presented with a seemingly insurmountable task in front of you? One that stands between you and your destiny? For me, that's how it felt. It was a mountain.

Finally, the day before the exam came. I downed as much caffeine as I could without giving myself too many palpitations and studied with all I had in me. I knew it was still not enough.

Have you experienced those times? Times where you gave it your all, and you still came up short?If you are in one of these moments, do not lose hope. God will meet you in your lowest valley. He will break through any barrier to help His child in need.

Well, that barrier was PDx for me. I went to bed that night disheartened. Actually, I was sick to my stomach. The only thing I had left to do was pray. Looking back now, I realize that should have been the first thing I did, not the last resort. Yet, sometimes we fall prey to the lies of the enemy. We miss the answer right in front of us.

That night, I prayed to God that if He wanted me to be a physician, then I was going to need His help. I was going to need a supernatural intervention for my lackluster brain power. He was going to have to step in and congeal all the facts in my head into an organisable heap.

I remember slipping off to sleep and feeling a sense of dread. I was definitely not counting sheep.

Sometime in the early morning hours, I had one of the most vivid dreams I have ever had. I was utterly exhausted, yet this dream was crystal clear. As I lay asleep, a teacher in front of a whiteboard came into view. I only saw their back. I didn't know who the teacher was, but I was more interested in what he was writing down. My attention was drawn to the board.

I saw him write one sentence after the next. Sentences that were questions. One after another. There were approximately 20 questions in total. I was asleep, but the clarity of my thoughts was far from that. My mind was at full attention.

After the last question was written, I was startled awake. As I was suddenly pulled from my dream back into reality, I heard the instructions, "*Write down what you saw.*" I rapidly searched my room, grabbed my notebook and pen and began feverishly writing down the images still burned into my brain.

One after another. Twenty questions gradually appeared on the page in front of me. Twenty questions that I was remembering from the dream.

This was now 4 o'clock in the morning. The time that I usually woke up on test days. Some would say it was a bit extreme to wake up that early, but I enjoyed the early mornings. They allowed me time to mainline some coffee and have time pouring over last-minute notes. Aka cramming. Yes, I know. I am not in favor of or recommending cramming, but I was going to do everything I could to pass this class.

As the minutes ticked by, the unusual morning session went on. The next thing I heard after finishing the questions was, "*Now, find the answers*". I complied. I rapidly went through my massive PDx packet and searched for the answers to these questions. It shockingly didn't take me too long. The questions were all ones that had been a large focus in the course. I just had not been present enough to wade through the course in the state I was in.

A few hours went by, and I was getting ready to sit for the exam. It was now 8 o'clock, and I was sitting at my desk. This was it. This was the final exam standing between me and becoming a second-year medical student. This was the moment where I found out if I would move forward or be held back.

Was I really going to be able to become a physician and fulfill the dream God had put on my heart?I prayed one more time and began the test. As the pages went by, I could barely believe what I was seeing. Every single one of the test questions I had seen in my dream was on the test. Every. Single. One. Not one was missing.

I don't think I have ever been so sure of passing a test as I was that day. I knew that I had remembered enough and had answered enough questions right that I was going to be moving on to the second year.

It was only a day later when I got the confirmation. I had

passed. God had come through in an unusual way. The Holy Spirit had broken through my weakness and my brokenness and had given me help to move forward into what He was calling me to do. I was on my way to fulfilling the calling God had placed on my life.

Some may be wondering if this type of experience was something that happened frequently for me. No. This was not my study tactic for the rest of my training in medical school. I never had another dream like I had that night. This was my launching point though. This was the night where God supernaturally stepped into my reality and gave me a nudge into my destiny.

From that day forward, I had to put in the work and keep pushing past what I believed I could do. But that moment was a turning point in my relationship with God. It was when the God of the Bible had become real to me. The God of Abraham, Isaac, and Jacob became the God of Emily.

It was a moment when I knew beyond a shadow of a doubt that unless He had intervened, I would not be where I am today.

These are the moments when God becomes real. These are the moments when you realize God can be trusted. He is the same yesterday as He is today and as He will be tomorrow. Once you truly understand this, your eyes will be opened.

He is good, and He is for you. Moments like these are where you go from head knowledge to heart knowledge.

Through the Noise

It was only a few years later that I had my next encounter with God. An encounter that was much more subtle. This time, He was drawing me in. He wasn't going to boldly burst through reality and show me the answer. No, He was asking me to lean in. He was having me know what it felt to sense the still, small voice.

Just like a radio station, when you first start hearing from the Holy Spirit, He will begin teaching you how to listen to Him. He will begin helping you tune into the right frequency. To cut out the other noise. To hear beyond the static.

Sometimes, God speaks to us in very subtle ways and other times, He is more clear. Sometimes, He will use shakings or earthquakes, sometimes wind and sometimes it will be a gentle whisper. He speaks in different ways because not all circumstances are the same. There are times when getting our attention may mean the difference between life and death.

The Bible is filled with examples of God speaking to his people in various ways. Times where He needed to get their attention. One of my favorite examples was when God spoke to Elijah when he was greatly discouraged. I guess this can happen when one has a crazy woman such as Jezebel threatening them. I'm sure you have experienced one or two of these in your life. Yes, I said it. And yes, I am a woman.

Well, this was an instance where the Lord spoke very clearly to his friend. He had Elijah come near so He could teach him that he was not alone. He had him come near because our God is the ultimate comforter.

"And he said, "Go out and stand on the mount before the Lord." And behold, the Lord passed by, and a great and strong wind tore the mountains and broke in pieces the rocks before the Lord, but the Lord was not in the wind.
And after the wind an earthquake, but the Lord was not in the earthquake.
And after the earthquake a fire, but the Lord was not in the fire.
And after the fire the sound of a low whisper. And when Elijah heard it, he wrapped his face in his cloak and went out and stood at the entrance of the cave. And behold, there came a voice to him and said, "What are you doing here, Elijah?"
1 Kings 19: 11-13 *ESV*

Isn't that like God? To ask us a question that He already knows the answer to?

He knew why Elijah was hiding, and He knows why you and I behave the way we do. He loves us anyway. Even in our weakness and in our dark places, He wants to connect with us so that His friendship can begin to transform us. To begin to prune off the dead areas and to show us ways where we are to come up higher.

Well, for me, the next time God really spoke to me, He needed me to come up much higher. Looking back, the next time I really heard from the Holy Spirit was in my 4th year of medical school. As I had mentioned, my life kind of fell apart during my medical school years. The healing after a divorce was not immediate, especially when I was mostly burying my head in the sand so I could make it through schooling. Although I was getting by scholastically at that point, every other area of my life was far from thriving. I numbed myself in all the wrong ways. To anyone who knew me during that time period, one would have referred to my life as a bit of a "dumpster fire".

I don't know if you have experienced deep hurt, but my pain did not bring out the best in me. I understand why divorce was never meant to be in God's original plan. The wave of devastation it can leave in its wake is very painful.

Well, as you may have guessed, I was the worst version of myself in medical school and in residency. I still loved God with all my heart but had allowed the hurt I experienced from divorce to seep into me and change me. I made a lot of poor choices.

That's the problem with spiritual roots. When not evaluated and appropriately dealt with, unseen things under the surface can influence things that are seen. Living with bitterness, anger, or unforgiveness will make its way to the surface, one way or another. Hurt people end up hurting others. I was no exception to this.

I look back on those years with regret. Although I have repented and am forgiven, I wish I could have saved myself and others the heartache that encompassed that period of time.

Well, in the midst of the tumultuous period of learning to do what God called me to do, He spoke again. It was now towards the end of medical school when I heard His voice again. I was at the start of my 4th year of medical school, and I was rapidly approaching an important decision. I was deciding which residency I would be applying for. Up until that time, I was undecided.

With each rotation I did in medical school, I seemed to get more unsettled in this decision. I would start each rotation with hope, but by the end of it, I would realize it was a poor fit. I couldn't see myself doing that specialty for a long time. What was I going to do? Time was running out.

Well, I finally rotated again in the Emergency Department. I realized by then that I had gained some knowledge as a medical student. I felt a tad less apprehensive that my lack of knowledge was going to immediately kill any patient walking through the doors of the ED.

By the end of the rotation, my mind was made up. I liked solving the puzzling cases that walked through the doors and liked having a wide range of people that I saw. I also loved how laid back the emergency medicine physicians seemed to be. They just seemed more like my people.

Now, the only issue was that Emergency Medicine was a difficult residency to match into. That is the thing as a medical student. You don't get to fully decide what specialty you are going to end up in as a physician. Yes, you did the training and got the degree but if you are not a competitive candidate, you may not be placed or *"match"* into a residency that allows you to become the type of physician you are wanting to become.

The thing about medical school is that all of the other students in your class are typically good candidates. The field has already been leveled, and those that couldn't handle it were already weeded out. So, you are up against the top of the top performers. That's the not-so-fun part of training.

How was I going to solve this issue of matching into my field? I was definitely concerned with the real possibility of not being able to match into this competitive field. I realized what stood between me and my new goal of becoming an emergency medicine physician was an away rotation. This would help my application to be more competitive. There was one main issue with this. Securing an away rotation.

What this meant was that I had to scramble to find a hospital somewhere in the country that had a rotation spot to teach me some basics of what it is like to work as an Emergency Medicine physician. These rotations are used to expose one further to the specialty to see if it is a good fit. The program has a chance to see who you are and how you work and the candidate has the chance to gain experience and knowledge. It is a win-win situation.

So, I buckled down and sent out applications to multiple programs across the US. The first one that responded was in a town named Manhasset on Long Island. I was elated when I heard that I would be going to New York! I had seen the shows. I thought I knew what I was in for.

The only issue now was finding housing. That can't be that hard, right? Well, the issue now was that I did not know of one single person who lived in New York. Not one. That was paired with the other issue of me being a broke student.

Like I said, I had watched the shows. I knew New York housing was not cheap. Especially for a 6-week rotation, yet I knew I needed to secure a spot.

By that time in my training, I had begun seriously dating another medical student. A really good guy that had started out as a friend and had become much more. I'm sure those around us could see the bigger picture of the relationship red flags, yet we were blind to them at that time.

He was someone who was a life raft for me during that

dark period. Unfortunately for him, I was not a life raft. I was quite the opposite. My state of mind and lack of healing from my divorce made me more like a siren that caused him to crash against a shore. Like I said earlier, hurting people hurt other people. I was no exception to this rule.

Looking back now, I wish I would have saved him the hurt. I wish he wouldn't have been a casualty. Yet, I had allowed the enemy to so completely destroy my identity and self-esteem that I believed that my worth came through my connection to another. That lie was a snare for both of us. That's the thing with lies about self-worth. They don't just affect the self. Others often get caught in the cross hairs.

Looking back now, I know my story would have been much different had he not been a large portion of one of my chapters. Although it was a tumultuous few pages, I am thankful for the lessons I learned in that period of time. I truly don't know if I would have made it through those years without a life raft. That's the thing with people who are part of our stories. They may not be there at the start or the end, but they are with us in the middle. When we experience turbulence along the way, God can bring blessing out of these darker places if we only let Him.

Well, when my boyfriend found out that I needed housing in New York, he immediately began working on a solution. It was not long before he found me a great place. The location seemed absolutely perfect. It was a multi-unit apartment that was right next to the water. There were 6 or 7 other female medical students who would also be at the apartment. I was excited! How could things get better than this for an away rotation?!

I thought it would be the perfect getaway to New York

while also learning about my new chosen specialty. It was perfect until a few weeks later when the dread set in. It started gradually at first. A sick feeling. A pit in the base of my stomach. You know the type. Knowing that something is wrong, but you can't fully decide why it is wrong. I could not shake the feeling.

As each day went by, it grew stronger and stronger. What was it? Why was I losing my peace? Why was I now dreading this "*perfect*" location?

Then it came, barely as a whisper. Looking back now, it mostly came as a knowing. I realized that the rotation itself was not causing this feeling, but I knew that I could not stay at this apartment. It was a knowing that is very difficult to explain. If you have ever experienced anything like this, then I'm sure you know what I am talking about. It is knowledge without knowing how you have the knowledge.

By now, I had enough of a track history with God that even though I did not understand why, I understood that I better listen to this feeling. To this prompting. That was it. I had made up my mind that I needed to change my housing. I wasn't given a reason. God was asking me to trust Him.

We often aren't given the answers to our toughest questions right away. That's the hard part about faith. It is trusting in the One who has the answers when we don't know what those answers fully are.

All I knew for sure that day was that I had no peace staying in the house near the beach. No peace accepting the opportunity that looked perfect on paper. The one that was full of worldly wisdom.

So, I spoke to my boyfriend again. I told him I was not comfortable with the housing. I told him that I wasn't sure why, but I was going to need to change my housing. He shockingly understood and didn't put up any resistance. He immediately began looking for other housing.

It wasn't much time before he found another opportunity. This one, however, did not seem so outwardly perfect. It was a chance to share an apartment with an OB-GYN resident who happened to be a man. We knew that this resident had a legitimate email address that corresponded with the residency program, but it was not the answer I had quite expected.

Staying with an unknown man who lived in an apartment I would be staying at was definitely not what I had pictured on my first getaway to New York. This was a person I had never met or spoken with and he lived in an apartment located in a city I had never visited. Looking back now, it most definitely seemed like the plot in a bad movie. One that did not go well for the woman.

The interesting part was that this scenario felt okay. There was no bad feeling associated with this decision. I immediately had total peace about it.

That's the thing when you are listening to God. Oftentimes, the decisions that make the least sense when looking at them through worldly vision make the most sense when looking at them through a kingdom lens.

That was this choice. Bad on paper but peaceful in my soul. I came to learn that this resident lived on campus, approximately 400 feet from the hospital where I would be working. I would no longer need to rent a car. I could walk to work.

I can't fully explain it but it just felt right. So, I signed the papers and prepared for my trip.

As I flew out for my rotation, I kept hearing alarming phrases on the news. These were words that sounded quite concerning, but ones I thought probably were said a lot on the East Coast. Once again, I thought I knew all I needed to know. I mean, I had watched the shows. However, this seemed a bit different. This time, I kept hearing warnings of a large hurricane. Surely, it was just another overblown media frenzy piece. One that gets you all riled up and fearful and happens to not really turn into anything significant. Like I said, west coast mentality and not in a great head space at that time.

Well, it was only a couple days after I landed in New York when I realized why the Holy Spirit had given me the firm instructions to change locations. It didn't take long to see what God was protecting me from.

The Storm

Hurricane Sandy hit, and it hit hard. It caused significant devastation in the area. It caused widespread power outages that lasted for weeks. It caused ridiculously long gas lines as people were frantically trying to find this commodity. It caused flooding and chaos in the exact area where I had originally planned on staying.

I still remember being holed up in that tiny, cozy apartment right next to the hospital as the winds howled outside my window. I was warm and comfortable with candles flickering while my friends and family were praying and fearing for my safety. The power went out for a short period of time, but I just stayed inside and remained comfortable.

I was acutely aware that it was the hand of God and the

still, small voice of the Holy Spirit who had warned me to avoid the apartment on the water. He had been the one who told me to seek another location that was next to the hospital. It was the Holy Spirit's urgings that allowed me to be spared from a building that I would have needed to be evacuated from.

I have thought many times since then, where would I have gone to? What would have happened if I had ignored that still, small voice?

It was the Holy Spirit that gave me supernatural instructions so I would be spared from losing power for 2-3 weeks during a cold season in New York. Instead, I was in apartments where the hospital personnel had priority to have the power restored so they could take care of the hurricane victims. I only lost power for half a day rather than half a month.

The Lord had spared me from staying in 2-plus hour gas lines as I had already given up my rental car as it was unnecessary to have one with my short walking commute. Not only was God keeping me safe, He was sparing me from the extra stress and time that would have potentially impacted that rotation.

When my parents called me, they were shocked at how peaceful I was. They were watching the news, and everything I told them was the exact opposite of what they were seeing. They barely believed their own daughter. The Holy Spirit had given me peace that surpassed understanding. He had given peace in the midst of a large storm, quite literally.

By the way, it was this same rotation that landed me my residency slot. That's the thing with God. He will work all things for good. What could have been a tragic rotation filled with stress and confusion ended up being one of the most relaxed time periods I had in New York. God doesn't always stop the storms from coming, but He does oftentimes send life rafts if we have eyes to see and ears that hear.

So, what does this story mean for you? Why am I telling you of a testimony of how the Holy Spirit moved in my life? Why am I telling you of two encounters with God? Because it is through encountering God that we become changed. That we begin to learn to trust Him. That we begin to know we can follow His lead.

Because it is by testimony that I can show you there is supernatural intelligence. You can have it if you open yourself up to His leading. This is not ordinary intelligence I am speaking of. It is knowledge that comes directly from the heart of the Father. It is by testimony that we can wake the others up.

The Holy Spirit is the same comforter, advisor and advocate to you as He is for me. He has all wisdom and all guidance and will literally show you which path to take. The key is that we need to be tuned in to His frequency. We must learn how He speaks. We need to see how He moves. We need to continually be seeking to walk with Him. Not ahead of Him. Not behind Him. But hand in hand. Daily with our decisions.

Just like we are with any of our closest friends. We learn their idiosyncrasies. We learn their patterns. We learn what their voice sounds like. We see patterns in how they move.

Are you ready to begin to tune in to these frequencies? If so, begin to look back on periods of time when you had a knowing that you shouldn't have had. Begin to ask the Holy Spirit to reveal times in your life where He went before you and protected you. Where He spoke to you and warned you of something that spared you heartache. Or times where you perhaps went ahead even against the warning. What was the outcome when you chose not to listen?

Take time to remember the moments where He was speaking to you in His still small voice or in dreams. These are your training wheels. These are the times where you are learning what it means to hear the voice of the Holy Spirit. Times where you are learning what it means to have a friendship with the King of the universe.

This King is still encountering you today. He wants to have a personal relationship with you. He is not after rules and legalism. He is not for religion. He is all about relationships. He loves you and is for you and He still speaks today.

Some may wonder if they can hear His voice. If this is you, ask yourself this question. Have you ever heard the hisses of doubt in your ears? Have you heard that you were not good enough, not smart enough, not pretty enough, etc? Well, if you can hear these lies of the enemy, you can encounter the Word of God. You can hear His voice. You can hear the voice that speaks Life, not death over you.

He will meet you wherever you are at. Sometimes, it will be in the earthquake. Sometimes, in the storm. And sometimes through the still, small voice.

Why is this such an important key for your life and your work? Because there will come a time when you will need to be so finely tuned in to this frequency that you must tune out all other noise. A time when the world grows dark. A time when you must unmistakably hear the still, small voice of your closest friend. It is in these moments that you will recognize His voice. The voice of the Holy Spirit.

I urge you today to take the time to tune in. Invest your time in growing close to the greatest friend you could ever ask for. Spend moments listening to what He has on His heart.

Encountering God is a key to reviving your own heart so you can revive the heart of medicine.

Loving Judas

"So now faith, hope, and love abide, these three; but the greatest of these is love."
1 Corinthians 13:13 *ESV*

Love is the second key to reviving the heart of medicine. Yet, it is not just any ordinary love that will cause a heart to beat again. No, something supernatural must take place. You can't act like the world if you are going to transform the world around you. This is going to require going way beyond worldly love. It is going to require your heart to beat differently than it is used to.

What do I mean by this statement? I am asking you to step out into an area that is not comfortable and one that does not come naturally. You are called to love the unlovable. You are called to love Judas. The one that betrayed you. Perhaps one who has broken you. Usually it is one who you feel is not worthy of love. The person you don't want to pray for and the one you hope you never see again.

Judas was a broken person. He was part of Jesus' inner circle. He started out as a friend who later betrayed Jesus for financial gain. Judas had some good qualities, yet he allowed the enemy to influence him to harm the one that he should have protected. If you are brutally honest, he is like you and me.

Statue of Unconditional Love

In a wide-open space at Loma Linda University, there stands a regal bronze-colored statue consisting of four very different men. These men were strangers before their paths crossed. They had never known one another before their story was immortalized in this special space.

These men were unaware that their story and actions would be one that has been spoken about for generations. They were unaware that their story would be one that has influenced the heart of my patients' care.

Even in my med student hustle days, these four characters would always catch my eye as I walked by them to class each morning. There were many times I caught myself staring at the scene. I didn't fully realize it at the time, but I was being caught up in the meaning of something much bigger than myself. I was always moved by this unchanging scene that seemed to speak a thousand words in a mere moment.

To this day, I still remember the first man standing in the scene. He is a priest. You can't mistake his appearance. He is wearing the typical flowy garb, and his head is adorned with an ostentatious beretta. He has a hardened look on his face, and he is fully turned away from the others in the scene. You can almost see the pride and disdain seeping out of his pores. Before you become offended, this is not about religion, it is about relationships. It is about one who turns away from those in need.

As you go on, you see another man. This one is not as heavily decorated as the first. He appears to also be wearing a flowy robe, but unlike the first one, he is wearing a much more underwhelming headpiece than the first man. You can tell he also holds some sort of station in the church, but he is less ornamented than the first.

This second man is looking down in shock at the final two men in the figure. He is doing nothing but holding his face, observing the dramatic scene right in front of him. You can see he has some internal turmoil that he should be doing something, but thoughts are clearly not producing action in this one.

Finally, you turn your gaze to the last two men in the scene. You see one who is sprawled out, his body in obvious agony. You see his mouth and eyes are closed, his deformed body hanging lifelessly over the other man. You see that this one cannot even lift his own head. His head is being held compassionately by a man who is on his knees. This final man in the scene is the true focus of the story. He is lovingly looking down at the injured man, and he shows love through his actions. He is the epitome of binding up the wounded and the broken hearted.

Have you seen this scene before, whether in your head or in person? Perhaps you have read about it? If you have ever opened your Bible then I believe you probably have. The fourth man in the scene is the Good Samaritan. He is the one whom Jesus spoke about in the following passage:

"On one occasion, an expert in the law stood up to test Jesus. "Teacher," he asked, "what must I do to inherit eternal life?"

"What is written in the Law?" he replied. "How do you read it?"

He answered, "'Love the Lord your God with all your heart and with all your soul and with all your strength and with all your mind'; and, 'Love your neighbor as yourself.'"

"You have answered correctly," Jesus replied. "Do this and you will live."

But he wanted to justify himself, so he asked Jesus, "And who is my neighbor?"

In reply Jesus said: "A man was going down from Jerusalem to Jericho, when he was attacked by robbers. They stripped him of his clothes, beat him and went away, leaving him half dead.A priest happened to be going down the same road, and when he saw the man, he passed by on the other side. So too, a Levite, when he came to the place and saw him, passed by on the other side. But a Samaritan, as he traveled, came where the man was; and when he saw him, he took pity on him.He went to him and bandaged his wounds, pouring on oil and wine. Then he put the man on his own donkey, brought him to an inn and took care of him.The next day he took out two denarii and gave them to the innkeeper. 'Look after him,' he said, 'and when I return, I will reimburse you for any extra expense you may have.'

"Which of these three do you think was a neighbor to the man who fell into the hands of robbers?"

The expert in the law replied, "The one who had mercy on him."
Jesus told him, "Go and do likewise."
Luke 10:25-37 *NIV*

If you are in healthcare, you are being told to go and do likewise. Even if you aren't in healthcare, you are called to be a Good Samaritan. You are called to help those in need. To help others who are less fortunate than you. To bind up the broken, not to be the one who is doing the breaking.

Every day, you must realize that you are making the choice to be one of these characters. Your actions show whether you are the one who is focused on your own priorities and so caught up in yourself that you do not have time to stop and lift others up or if you are someone who has compassion on others. One who puts aside their selfish ambitions and takes time to lift another up.

If you are the first character, you are the one who believes another one's pain is not your problem. Your heart does not beat for others. No matter what is going on around you, it is easy for you to go about your day per usual. You have things to do, people to see, places to go. You are always on a mission, but not a mission to help others.

Perhaps you aren't as cold as the first man. Maybe you are the second character. The one who does feel a bit of pity for others. The one who is looking at the situation and looking at the pain but doesn't really feel like it's your responsibility to do anything about it. I mean, there are others who are around. Clearly, someone else can fix that problem. You have things to do. It's a nice thought to help others, but you are so busy. You must be about your business. You have so many church meetings to attend or duties at your job that taking the time to help the less fortunate infringes on how you think your day should go.

This type of person is one who doesn't like to ruffle feathers. You know, it's best to go with the flow. You don't like to make a scene. You don't want to stand out. With this mindset, you are someone who isn't willing to stand for something, which makes you easy prey to fall for anything.

It is the lack of love in action that keeps pews empty in a church. The lack of focus that keeps decade-long Christians asleep at the wheel of life and makes a provider one who is a clinician only. Not a healer. It is a focus based on mere words rather than on the loving actions our Savior has asked us to do. Christianity that does not take action is not Christianity at all. We must be good soil and produce fruit.

Open your eyes to assess your actions. You don't have to stay as the first two characters in that story. My hope and prayer is that you are the loving character in the scene. That you are or strive to be the Good Samaritan. The one on whom the scene is focused. The one that not only feels love and compassion for his fellow man, but one who chooses to act on these emotions. A person who chooses to help others even when it hurts. A human who chooses to have the heart of God. A clinician that shows God's love to patients each and every single day.

The Good Samaritan is a picture of an advocate. The Holy Spirit is the one who allows us to be an advocate for others. He is the one who helps us to love the unlovable.

Let me tell you a secret, though. No one is perfect at this. There are times when each one of us fails. I have failed many times. Honestly, it is typically when I have been frustrated when I was super tired or overworked. Perhaps offended. I failed to show love because I became focused on the wrong things. But that doesn't mean that you and I don't pick ourselves back up and work harder to love the unlovable. To show love and help others even when it hurts. Even when it personally costs.

My father, Wilfred Eastman Jr., MD, is a Good Samaritan physician. So was my grandfather. They taught me what it was like to stand in love for those around me. My dad taught me what it looked like to raise my voice and fight for my patients. He taught me that my priority should always lie first in what was best for my patient. Not what was best for myself.

He showed through his actions what it looked like to not always be popular in the eyes of many yet to be truly loved by those who were in his care. He taught me what hard decisions looked like when they were focused on love for God and for others. Is he perfect? No. Far from it. Just like all of us. Yet, he showed me what it looked like to love others even when they had directly hurt him.

My friend, Dr. B, who I introduced you to early in the book, was also a Good Samaritan physician. He always put himself on the line to help others. He stepped out and went above and beyond any time it meant he would be helping a hurting person. Although he is no longer with us, his short career was more meaningful than many others who have practiced for 30-plus years.

Jeffrey Evans, DO, is another mentor and a Good Samaritan physician. He taught me what it meant to be an emergency medicine physician who cared more about patients than about their throughput in the department. He showed me what it meant to practice patient care with the perspective of seeing my patients as my family and friends. Caring for them as I would want to be cared for.

When we are running on empty and are not being filled up with God's love, it is easy to forget the basics. To get distracted by the noise. We must consider that the length of our career is less important than the lasting impact we had on patients that God sent across our path. We must realize that the impact of a Good Samaritan physician always lives on in the hearts of their loved ones, along with those they worked with and those they cared for.

All of these life stories shaped my story and my practice of medicine. God gave me great examples that were meant to be a light to my path.

You and I are called to walk in those footsteps. We are called to bind up others' wounds as we go about our days. We are called to be a light. To truly love the unlovable and do the unthinkable. We must show love in action.

Loving Judas

Loving others is one of the greatest keys you will use when working in healthcare. But you must take it one step further. Loving Judas is the key to loving the unlovable. Loving Judas will be your biggest test and your greatest reward.

What do I mean by this? Judas was the disciple who betrayed Jesus. He was the one who betrayed the God of the universe for 30 pieces of silver. He sold out his mentor and friend for worldly gain. Spoiler alert. It was only a short-lived gain. He hung himself shortly after he betrayed his maker.

As I mentioned earlier, Judas was part of the inner circle. He was with Jesus, day in and day out of his years of ministry. He witnessed Jesus' love. He witnessed the miracles he performed. Yet, he betrayed our Lord into the hands of the high priests. Into the hands of the ones who would viciously beat him and place his body on a cross. People who were focused on religion, not relationships.

Judas was a person who was influenced and overtaken by the enemy. He was a key portion in Jesus' story and in our story of redemption.

Let's take things one step further. Take a moment to let this sink in and marinate as you grow more uncomfortable. Who is your Judas?

Judas is the person who has been the perceived villain in your story. The one who makes you cringe when you hear them spoken about. The one who hurt you when you helped them. The one who spreads lies about you. Perhaps the one who did something even more unspeakable to you. Judas is the hardest person that you will ever learn to love. Yet, loving Judas is one of the greatest keys to reviving the heart of medicine.

Personally, it has been the most challenging key for me to grab hold of. Let me explain. Almost a decade ago, I had someone come into my life who I perceived to be a Judas. Someone who, at every twist and turn, seemed to bring drama any time we interacted. Someone who I could not get away from, one who just really made life less than enjoyable.

Is anyone in your life coming into focus right now? Perhaps you are saved more than I am, and you don't have a

Judas. But some of you know what I'm talking about and know the type. To be fair, I'm sure I was the Judas in their story as well. That's the thing in these situations. There are always two sides to every story and two hearts that are often hurting. But since this is my story, I am sharing things from my perspective.

Regarding my Judas, whether it was finances that they were creating issues with, schedules, harsh comments, along with many other irritating things, it seemed impossible for me to see them through God's eyes. I struggled daily to keep myself from saying hurtful words when I felt cornered or hurt once again. Sometimes, I won the battle of taming my tongue, and other times, I lost it. The issue, though, was not with my tongue. It was a heart issue. I literally did not have any love in my heart towards them. I tried, but I just could not envision a future where I could love them.Yes, I know. It is sad.

I am sure, though, that I am not the only one who has dealt with this. Many Christ followers have felt betrayed by other Christ followers. I am sure that there are moments where your thoughts need to be redeemed. Moments where you need more than just a renewing of the mind. These are the times you need a renewing of your heart. This was definitely the case for me. I knew the lack of love in my heart was not right, but I did not know how to change. I had felt so wounded by them; I did not know how things could possibly be redeemed.

Yet, God kept working on me. He continually works to refine us with whatever means necessary to shape us into who He calls us to be.

God did not leave us there in that broken place. No, He

kept at it. Slowly, very slowly, chipping away the icy exterior and layers of the hurts over the years. It started first with a message of forgiveness. God speaking clearly one weekend that my husband and I were to forgive the one person who had made life very difficult for us. I could hardly believe it, but God was asking us to rise higher. He was asking us to be peacemakers. He was not okay leaving us in that pigpen wallowing in the mud. He kept after us. I slowly realized, even in my stubbornness, that He wasn't going to let this go. He kept showing word after word and working nonstop to soften our hearts.

It was on a cabin trip where He clearly spoke to us about what we needed to lay down if we were going to truly follow His lead. In our most favorite place that we love to visit. Our happy place: Greensprings Inn and Cabins. This was the place my husband and I would get away to reset and enjoy the bliss of each other's presence. This was the place that represented who we were as a couple. In love, enjoying the great outdoors and focusing on God and each other. It is fitting that the healing would begin in our happy place.

This trip was different, though. It had a mission. I didn't realize that God had set us up. Starting out the weekend, I had obsessively listened to a sermon series about Joseph. I could not stop listening to the biblical story of the favored son of Rachel, who was a dreamer. Due to unwarranted favor by his father and Joseph's own uncontrolled tongue, I listened as his brothers threw him into a pit. It was this pit that was his first stop on his way to his destiny in the palace.

The pastor discussed the pit, the prison, a palace and everything in between. He discussed Joseph's God-given ability to miraculously reveal the meaning of dreams. He discussed how God used this gift to save a nation.

It was at the cabin that we heard the pastor bring to life the fact that we must pass certain tests if we are going to fulfill the call of God in our life. We must go through these challenging seasons and learn to rise above the snares of the enemy. There is no way around these mountains, only through.

It was this series that refocused our vision of who we wanted to be individually and as a couple. It's not enough to be a gutless Christian who is merely biding time waiting for our Savior to return. No, we are to bring healing in the waiting. That weekend we learned that we must release those who have hurt us. Forgive those who broke us. Love those who hate us.

It was this series that was a scalpel to my heart. An incision that dissected away all the nastiness that I had concealed in my heart that was not allowing it to beat correctly. It was this sermon series and the promptings of the Holy Spirit that spoke clearly to my husband and me that we needed to write a letter. Not just any letter. We needed to write a letter to a person who had been a Judas in our story. To the one who had made a choice to betray and one who had inflicted pain on both of us over the past several years.

This letter was a key to unlocking our next chapter. It was a key that opened our eyes to the true poison of unforgiveness and the damage it causes when left unchecked. It was our first stop bringing us up from the pit.

Honestly, it was such a freeing letter to write. One that should have been written years before then. As we wrote, we thought we were freeing a prisoner. When we finished, it was our own hands that were being removed from the bars of our self-made prison cell. God used paper to begin to rewrite our story. He used a letter to move us forward to our destiny.

From that day forward, there was a subtle shift that began to take place. Releasing the poison of unforgiveness began to release the stranglehold the enemy had on my heart. That was just the beginning, though. As time went on, God gave me new vision. A new way to see that person through His eyes.

He began showing me that the ways they were acting really had nothing at all to do with me. He taught me that when they were doing things that were rude or annoying, it was not truly them that was behind those actions. It was the enemy working through them to inflict wounds.

He reminded me that the goal of the enemy was to kill, steal and destroy. He does not do that dressed in a costume with a pitchfork and a pointy tail. He works through people. He works through systems. He works through you and me. Hurt people will hurt other people. That saying is pure gold. That is a truth you must learn if you are to see your Judas through new eyes.

Once I began to truly see it was not them I was at war with, but it was the enemy of both our souls, that was the key to the prison break. That was when things really began to click.

As time went by, the emotions greatly eased. I was becoming a new person. My heart was being revived. The enemy was losing his grip in that situation. I could speak of the person in a normal manner and actually not be upset anymore. I even began to feel sadness and compassion at times. It continued on this level until the day we got the phone call. It was a phone call that rocked our family's world.

In a moment, my heart was broken for them. In a split second, my eyes were opened to the inordinate pain that person was experiencing. The pain that was now forever part of their story. I went from struggling to love them to realizing they needed all the love they could get. In an instant, I went from praying for my family to praying for the person who had just lost their world.

In an instant, it was no longer a difficult choice. It was like a shock from a defibrillator. My heart was fully reset. What a shock it is when we are snapped out of our selfish stories and our hearts are broken for another. What a feeling that comes over you when you realize the stupid and petty things you used to worry about are just that. They are stupid and petty.

This is a key that I didn't even realize I was missing. In this person's life, I was not being a Good Samaritan. I realized that when we are caught up in not loving others, we are unwittingly playing the first character in the Good Samaritan story. We are hardening our hearts with pride as we turn our faces. When we do this, we look away from the people that need our help the most. The ones that are the hardest to love are the ones that need the most love.

I don't care how long you have been a Christian. You have struggled with this at one time or another.

If you are in the healthcare field, you have run across a few Judas'. You have dealt with people who have spread lies about you, who may have belittled you, whose hearts are hardened and lacking in love. They hurt you and it was not good but don't let the pain keep you in this place. I am asking you to remember that love never fails. Love can find even the tiniest crack to go through. It can bring light even in the darkest of nights. It can transform any atmosphere.

Learning to love Judas is the key to loving the unlovable. Realizing the works of the enemy opens your eyes to seeing them with a new vision. As Paul so eloquently said,

"Love is patient and kind; love does not envy or boast; it is not arrogant or rude. It does not insist on its own way; it is not irritable or resentful; it does not rejoice at wrongdoing but rejoices with the truth. Love bears all things, believes all things, hopes all things, endures all things."
1 Corinthians 13:4-7 *ESV*

In an instant, your life can change. In an instant, your heart can be split wide open. Your dry and cracked heart can begin to beat with love for those who you never thought you would be able to love and care for.

Your patients are the same way. They are human, just like you and I. Your patients also need this message. They need your love. Your most difficult patients are hurting people. The ones who drive you crazy are the ones that need the most love.

It is hard. It is work. But do not turn your face away from them. Do not turn your face from those who need your love. Do not turn your face from those God created. The ones He chose to come across your path.

To transform the current culture of medicine, we are going to need to lay down many things. One of these things we will have to lay down is holding onto anger and hatred for those who have hurt us. We are going to have to dodge the arrows and look at the wounds they left. We must see the wounds so we can bind up the brokenhearted.

We cannot do this on our own. We must go to the One who has the power to redeem all circumstances. We must fully seek after the One who has the power to heal all hearts. He is the One who can help you love again. He is the key to helping you love your Judas so that you can be the Good Samaritan to all those who come across your path.

Loving Judas is a key to reviving the heart of medicine. God's love is the key to carrying the Heart of the Good Samaritan.

Relentless Courage

"They triumphed over him by the blood of the Lamb and by the word of their testimony; they did not love their lives so much as to shrink from death."
Revelation 12:11 *NIV*

This verse is the key to living and overcoming life as a follower of Christ. It is also a key to advancing the kingdom in medicine and shifting the atmosphere around us. As such, it is a main key I want to highlight on the journey to rising higher in our calling.

One cannot revive the heart of medicine without discussing the courage that is needed to do our jobs every single day. Not only courage, but persistence and courage. Being willing to stand up, no matter the cost for our patients. Being willing to not give up even in the face of insurmountable odds.

Let me be clear, these traits are not possible without Him. It is only with a renewing of our mind, and a reflection of His character that we can be a true advocate to those entrusted to our care. It is not a small task that is being required of us. People entrust us with their lives every single day.

As workers in the ministry of healing, we are not only called to be bold but we are called to be advocates. We are called to overcome by the sacrifice that Jesus willingly gave along with the word of testimony. It is only by looking to Him that we are given the skills and ability to act as His hands and feet in our daily lives. In the lives of our patients.

As the body of Christ and those who are working with the broken, working with those in their darkest moments to help restore health, we must realize that this responsibility comes with great sacrifice. If we are to mirror Christ's actions when walking with our patients, then we are going to need to rely on a power much greater than human will and strength to accomplish this purpose.

Christ alone is able to renew us. The true advocate of our souls is the only advocate who can teach us to follow in his steps. He has sent the Holy Spirit to help you do this.

So, what does it look like to live out advocacy in action? Advocacy that does not back down but instead persists against all odds. Let me show you. Remember Dr. B.? Well, this testimony will reveal to you who he truly was in the life of one patient and the life of his colleagues. A patient who had no clue how many events God lined up to save their life from teetering off the edge.

I remember the day very clearly. Yet, when I woke up that morning, I didn't realize how important that day would be. It's funny how we never fully know when Heaven is about to invade Earth. I didn't comprehend how that day would forever impact how I would see God's brilliance in timing, in bringing together a team for His purpose and showing me the meaning of advocacy in the face of extreme pressure.

That morning, I arrived at the hospital a bit later than usual. I wasn't actually the emergency medicine attending on shift. I wasn't the one in charge of seeing patients. Rather than walking into the ED, I walked through those double doors and walked to my admin office.

I had only been working on my paperwork for a couple of hours when I heard an overhead page. "*Trauma activation, 5 minutes*" – The sound of these words blaring overhead always filled me with apprehension. They repeated a similar jarring phrase overhead a second time just as the patient arrived.

Unlike many ED physicians who live for the rush and excitement, I was not one of the ED docs who lived for these moments. No, I always knew that the unexpected could happen. I always knew that I did not know everything in the world of medicine (as no physician truly does). I had learned in my time doing Emergency Medicine that it was these announcements that were my personal cue to begin praying. To seek heavenly wisdom to be able to help this person who was about to roll through the ambulance bay doors into the bright lights of our trauma room.

This time, though, I was not the person who was running the trauma. I was in the admin office, and I was just curious. Unusually curious. Something different was activated in me that day when I heard the overhead page. All I felt was curiosity. Interest in all the details of what this trauma could be. I wondered who was going to be rolling through the doors any moment. It was this curiosity that got me out of my roller chair and prompted me to walk down to the ED.

As I flashed my badge to open the doors, I walked to the trauma bay. Peering through the glass doors, I saw a skilled team working together, quick movements being completed, and orders being given in rapid succession. To some, this scene would appear chaotic. But to an ED doc, it is a classic and ordered scene where a team is working together to save a patient's life that hangs in the balance. A scene where every second matters. A chaotic but organized dance.

Quick decisions must be made, and the right actions must be taken. The key being in the right order. In a trauma, a systematic approach must be taken. One cannot miss any steps, as that could mean missing crucial details.

Working quickly to transfer the patient onto the trauma gurney, the team members knew their duties. There was one in scrubs who was placing the patient on cardiac leads and one starting a large bore IV. Another was taking a manual blood pressure. A respiratory therapist was standing in the corner just observing, waiting to see if the airway of the patient needed protection and waiting on the order for an EKG. The attending physician, one of my friends, was at the head of the bed running the show. He was calm and maintained his composure as he was the director of this trauma team.

I was always impressed with Dr. D. He was always cool under pressure. He was seasoned. He had seen much more than I.

As the patient returned from the CT scanner, I went back to review the images with Dr. D. Out of my mouth, I blurted the words, *"Looks like a burr hole is in order"*. I laughed a little nervously as I finished the sentence. Dr. D and I looked at each other. We both knew that the words were true.

For those who are not accustomed to the chaotic life in the ED or in an operating suite, a burr hole is a procedure very rarely done in the Emergency Department. It is so rare that most ED physicians never have to do one as an attending. These are procedures that used to be more common in tiny rural hospitals with no access to a neurosurgeon. They are taught to us as a medical student in the rare case we may one day need to know how to do this. They are procedures that one hopes never to have to use. Did I happen to mention we were in a tiny rural hospital without a neurosurgeon?

Well, going back to the burr hole. This is a procedure that involves using a drill to break through the hard exterior of the skull to allow drainage of blood from an underlying collection of blood. Basically, blood collects on the outer portion of one of the layers or meninges covering the brain. This procedure is one that is only used in a severe emergency when there are no other options. A lifesaving procedure that is only done when life is truly hanging in the balance.

Well, as I mentioned before, we were in a tiny rural hospital, and the closest neurosurgeon was over an hour away. We were living the scenario that we had trained several years ago for when working on cadavers. Except this time, there was a live person who had placed their utmost trust in us. One that needed our help.

Dr. D had concern in his voice when he told me the

patient was beginning to show neurological signs of herniation. Due to the severity of the injuries, he had already intubated the patient (placed her on a ventilator) shortly after arrival, but her pupils were showing less responsiveness when prompted by light.

This is a big deal. This means that pressure is so increased in the skull that nerves are beginning to lose function, and reflexes are being lost. It is only a matter of time before the patient's condition will be irreversible.

Well, Dr. D was a smart clinician, and he knew that a burr hole was in order, and I knew deep down that it was going to happen. We both knew that if we were going to do this, it was going to take both of us to have the courage to do something we were both scared to do. We didn't discuss this out loud. We just knew.

I hadn't told Dr. D that I had gotten extra training in neurosurgery when I was a medical student. I hadn't told him that Ben Carson's testimony in "*Gifted Hands*" was one of the main reasons I went into medicine. I hadn't told him that I had almost chosen neurosurgery as a career before I switched to emergency medicine. All I told him was that I had done a couple of burr holes about 7 years earlier.

Looking back now, I realize that God had put this moment in my heart almost a decade in advance of this patient encounter. I didn't know it at the time, but God knew there was a person who would need our help years down the road. God was going ahead of me. He was going before this patient. He was here with us.

So, we did what any logical and thorough ED physicians would do. As we had staff find the equipment to do the burr hole and begin setting the room up for this procedure, we began making phone calls. As we had nurses hanging hypertonic saline to try to lower the pressure in the brain and raise the head of the bed up to make sure to do everything we could to keep the patient safe, we were rapidly seeking help.

The first call was to ask a neurosurgeon to help walk us through the procedure. We knew our limitations but also knew they were the truly skilled surgeon who had done many of these before. We were ED physicians. We accepted the fact that their skill surpassed ours when it came to any procedure on the brain.

What we heard next shocked us. Dr. D heard the neurosurgeon's voice on the phone. He firmly instructed him, "*Do not do the burr hole. Ship the patient to my hospital*".

Dr. D was shocked. He went on. He kept explaining the severity of the patient's condition and that they would not make it to the hospital without herniating (becoming "*brain dead*"). The surgeon firmly stood his ground and said he could not recommend us doing the procedure. Now Dr. D was deflated.

When Dr. D told me this, I was not only shocked but I became angry. Something came over me, and I said, "*Try again. Call another hospital.*" There was something urging me to not give up. It was growing stronger and more stubborn by the moment. This patient had no family here to advocate for her life. We were it. We were the advocates.

So, this time, I made the phone call. I called a large tertiary hospital several hours away. I had spoken many times to their staff, and they were usually very helpful. I thought surely they would give us the answers and the blessing to complete the procedure. I spoke with the first neurosurgeon and then a second. One that was a fellow (still in training), and another was the attending (the final authority). Both said the exact same thing as the first neurosurgeon. They said, "*no.*" They said they could not recommend that we do the procedure.

My heart sank. I got off the phone and looked at Dr. D. We both knew that neither of us became doctors to watch our patients die in front of our eyes. We didn't go into a line of work to save lives just to have our hands tied when the moment came to save a life. We weren't going to accept defeat. We were going to learn what it meant to be an advocate when it mattered most.

I took a moment and contemplated our next move. I remembered my father's example so many times during his long career as an orthopedic surgeon. I remembered how many times he had fought against adversity to advocate for his patients. I thought about times where he would make the unpopular choice if it meant the right outcome.

I thought about this current situation and the certainty of a poor outcome for this patient if we did nothing. I realized that we were making a permanent decision that could either bring life or death. We could be ones that promoted healing or choose to be bystanders of her death. I realized quickly that I could only live with one option.

I took a deep breath and then looked Dr. D squarely in the eye and said, "*As the director of this department, I will sit on the stand with you and take the blame if this goes badly. I will be held just as responsible for going against the surgeon's advice. I give you my word on this.*" So, we both looked at each other a moment longer and he said, "*let's call the family. They are driving to the hospital right now.*"

So, Dr. D got on the phone and told the patient's loved

one to pull over. He needed them to park on the side of the road so they could clearly understand what we were saying to them. The gravity of what we were asking of them. This conversation mattered.

He explained the situation and told them that three neurosurgeons had told us we were not to do the burr hole procedure. He went on. He emphasized to the patient's loved one that both of us felt that was the wrong recommendation and the wrong conclusion. We were honest and straightforward. We knew we were outnumbered in opinion, but we were also the only physicians standing in front of the patient and we believed we must intervene if they had any hope of seeing their family member whole on this side of eternity.

The family member took a breath and said, *"Go ahead. Do everything you can for them."*

As Dr. D got off the phone, actions quickly unfolded. We rapidly moved to the head of the bed and began cutting through the tissues. We remembered the radiologist's voice and his recommendation to *"go high"*. To aim for a specific area where there was the most blood.

By this time, a crowd had gathered. People were showing up from other departments to see what crazy procedure they had heard we were doing. Many had never seen this procedure performed as we were only a tiny hospital. People showed up to root for an outcome that seemed impossible.

It was through this crowd that Dr. B walked. I still remember standing in my black stiletto heels doing a burr hole (yes, I told you it was an admin day!) as he walked into the trauma bay. I sensed movement in the corner of the room and briefly looked up.

He grinned and said, *"I heard you guys were doing something crazy... and having fun without me. What can I do to lend a hand?"*. That was Dr. B. Always one to help a patient or a colleague out. Always one who would go the extra mile.

You must realize what these words did to our courage. They were words of encouragement that were desperately needed. Ones that brought hope and helped us realize we had made the right choice. You must remember that a colleague's words can either give you courage or they can deepen your doubt. Words from one you trust can either bring life or death. Take time to stop and think the next time you want to give someone a piece of your mind. Are you going to be a healer or are you going to cause harm?

I still remember feeling the relief flood over both Dr. D and myself. We knew we had a surgeon who was bold enough to stop what he was doing to help us and the patient out. Dr. B went on to say that he had specifically trained at UCLA and was comfortable setting up a drainage system to evacuate the blood once we broke through the skull.

He knew he was not the one on call, and that didn't matter to him. He knew there was a patient who needed help and colleagues who were doing everything they could to save her. He was not going to miss out on an opportunity to save a life. And, true to his word, as we broke through the skull and realized we had completed the burr hole, Dr. B went to work. He set up a J-tube drain and began rapidly evacuating the blood that was pressing the patient's brain down into the base of the skull. Moments went by, and we saw that he was successfully draining the blood. We knew that we had done what we could. Now we waited.

The patient remained on the ventilator and remained

sedated. We saw no changes as the EMS crew came to package her up to bring her to the larger hospital with the services she needed. Only time would tell if our efforts made any difference in the life of this patient.

We shipped the patient off to the first neurosurgeon's hospital. Yes, the one who had been the first to tell us not to complete the procedure. Gulp. That was quite a long transfer for both Dr. D and myself. We waited. Then we waited some more.

I can tell you with certainty the pressure I felt in my bones from this experience was great. I can tell you this pressure was more intense than any I had ever felt while practicing medicine. It was the kind that caused the ball in your throat to feel as if it had a chokehold on you and the knot in your stomach to feel like you were going to vomit.

We waited some more. So much time went by that I ended up going home. Rattled. I prayed. Prayed for the patient and prayed for protection.

I remember being in my living room when I got the call. A call from Dr. D. He told me that the neurosurgeon had called him. He said that when he answered the phone, the surgeon asked a leading question. One that made his heart palpitate. *"Are you the physician who went against my recommendation and did a burr hole?"*

He said *"Yes. I am one of two."*

The neurosurgeon paused and said, *"Thank you. Thank you for going against my recommendation."* Gulp. He went on, *"I have repeated the patient's CT scan, and all blood has been removed. I could not have done a better job. Now we wait to see how they respond."*

Those of you who have worked in the field of medicine

know that this conversation was the second miracle of the day. Both Dr. D and I felt the breath return to our own lungs.

We laughed hysterically as he told me that this conversation almost made him soil his pants. I didn't tell him at that time, but it almost made me do that too. I mean, I am a lady. I'm not supposed to say those things typically, especially when wearing heels. But to be clear, I was considering my options for clothing changes.

The moment that really mattered though, came 4 months later. The patient, who had been the star of the trauma show, walked through those glass double doors. Did you hear that?! She walked through those doors on her own two feet. She had gone through months of grueling rehab, but she was upright and talking. She was on a mission to thank the team that had risked it all to save a life.

God had spared her life, and she knew it. We knew it. Looking back, I realized how much God had done that day. How many things had He lined up? How long had He been working to save this life?

God had not only been working that day for our patient. He had found three physicians from different walks of life to save a life. He had lined up our shifts and routines that day so that we could be the hands and feet of Christ. He had put a fire in all our hearts to not stand idly by and watch life pass on. No. He told each one of us to come up higher.

He told us to go against all odds and recommendations. He invited us to have the courage to fight for our patient so we could be part of His work in healing her. He emboldened us not to shrink back but told us instead to advance forward as advocates. He gave us the boldness to be his hands and feet that day.

Advocacy. This is what we are called to do. This is who we are called to be. Courage. This is what we need to possess to be a team that heals patients. Not in moments when the lights are on and we are on a stage. No, in the quiet moments, too.

As healthcare workers, we are to stand in the gap. We are to fight for our patients, no matter the cost. We are not to go against laws or break rules; however, there are times that we must look from a higher vantage point and see what is really at stake.

If we had let the fear of the neurosurgeon overwhelm us, we would have panicked and stopped. We would have stayed on the ground, and the patient would not have recovered.

If we had focused on what could be the potential outcome of things not going well and the family coming against us, the patient would not be present with us today. If we would have kept our eyes focused on the waves, we would have surely sunk.

So today, I am calling you up higher.

I don't know if you are a nurse. Perhaps you are a family practice physician. Maybe you are a nurse practitioner or a physician's assistant. Or even a neurosurgeon. It does not matter your title. It matters what you do with that title.

You are not to settle when things get tough. You are called to be an advocate. You are called to fight for what is in the best interests of your patient, not to settle for your comfort zone.

You were created to step up and not back down. You are

called to be Christ to your patients. To move with His Spirit, not the spirit of the world.

You think this is a big ask? A big calling? That's right. It is. It's time to put on your big boy pants or perhaps your strappy stilettos. Those who are called higher are the ones that shift atmospheres. They are the ones who are not willing to stay on the ground. They seek Him and His wisdom and move forward, through the fear.

So, get ready. It's time to soar. Get ready to boldly step forward and be the advocate for others that you would want them to be for you. Get ready to be the change that you want to see in medicine.

As you step forward, remember these words. Take time to meditate on them:

"Speak up for those who cannot speak for themselves, for the rights of all who are destitute. Speak up and judge fairly; defend the rights of the poor and needy."
Proverbs 31:8-9 *NIV*
"Is not this the kind of fasting I have chosen; to loose the chains of injustice and untie the cords of the yoke, to set the oppressed free and break every yoke?"
Isaiah 58:6 *NIV*

Declare these words over yourself and your family. Pray for God to not only use you but to make you usable. You have what it takes as long as you are connected to the One who makes all things possible. Through Him, you are more than able.

God is calling you to be courageous today. He is calling

you to persist in the face of doubt. Have the courage today to step out in faith and watch Him use you to revive the hearts of those around you!

Peace. Be Still

"Peace I leave with you; my peace I give you. I do not give to you as the world gives. Do not let your hearts be troubled and do not be afraid."
John 14:27 *NIV*

Have you ever known someone whose presence brought peace to you? One who was calm and steady even when all hell was breaking loose around them? The type of person who stays collected and thinks well under pressure. The one that can keep their eyes focused on the task, no matter the distraction.

Well, if you are in healthcare, you are called to be that person. You are called to bring peace even in the most chaotic of situations. Your patient's lives depend on this quality. Your colleagues are counting on you to be calm. You must be steady even with the waves crashing against you.

You were created to do this. You can do this. You can be the one used to shift the wind, the waves and the storm. But here's the key. You are not the one who is actually bringing peace and calming the storm. You are the messenger He is working through. Let me explain.

Remember the night when the disciples were told to cross the sea of Galilee? The time that Jesus told them to go to the other side. It was on a very dark night when you watch seasoned fishermen realize they did not have peace in every storm.

"That day when evening came, he said to his disciples, "Let us go over to the other side." Leaving the crowd behind, they took him along, just as he was, in the boat. There were also other boats with him.A furious squall came up, and the waves broke over the boat, so that it was nearly swamped.Jesus was in the stern, sleeping on a cushion. The disciples woke him and said to him, "Teacher, don't you care if we drown?"
He got up, rebuked the wind and said to the waves, "Quiet! Be still!" Then the wind died down and it was completely calm. He said to his disciples, "Why are you so afraid? Do you still have no faith?"
Mark 4:35-40 *NIV*

We can relate to those in the boat. Can you feel the sheer terror? Can you sense what they must have been thinking? While Jesus was sleeping and at complete peace, they were seeing the wind and the waves. They knew that their boat did not stand a chance. They were looking at the facts and missing the Truth.

They were not at peace, but they carried peace. They carried the Prince of Peace in that boat. Why did they miss this fact? Because they were so distracted by the storm in their life that night, they lost the truth. Their reality was viewed through a lens of terror as they had not yet learned they carried the Authority to calm the wind and the waves.

From our vantage point, we know that the storm never stood a chance against the One who has the power to calm the wind and the waves. If only the disciples knew what they carried. They fell for facts when they should have been seeking the Truth. They carried their Lord and Savior in that boat. They had the answer right there with them but they needed a revelation of who He truly was.

The funny thing is this was only their first water lesson. Jesus was going to have them do a repeat round with the gale-force winds and the storm-battering waves. This time, though, He was going to witness how much they had learned from the first test. He had given them an open book test the first-time round, and now they were going to have to step out in what He had taught them. This time, the teacher was going to remain silent and watch from afar.

The start of the next water lesson was quite similar. It again involved Jesus telling them to go to the other side of the lake. This time, however, He sent them ahead of him to the other side. He was going to stay alone to pray and spend time with the Father. They were sent on ahead, but they had no clue they were headed into their next storm.

Their test was just beginning...

"Immediately Jesus made the disciples get into the boat and go on ahead of him to the other side, while he dismissed the crowd. After he had dismissed them, he went up on a mountainside by himself to pray. Later that night, he was there alone, and the boat was already a considerable distance

from land, buffeted by the waves because the wind was against it.

Shortly before dawn Jesus went out to them, walking on the lake. When the disciples saw him walking on the lake, they were terrified. "It's a ghost," they said, and cried out in fear. But Jesus immediately said to them: "Take courage! It is I. Don't be afraid."

"Lord, if it's you," Peter replied, "tell me to come to you on the water."

"Come," he said.

Then Peter got down out of the boat, walked on the water and came toward Jesus. But when he saw the wind, he was afraid and, beginning to sink, cried out, "Lord, save me!" Immediately Jesus reached out his hand and caught him. "You of little faith," he said, "why did you doubt?"

And when they climbed into the boat, the wind died down. Then those who were in the boat worshiped him, saying, "Truly you are the Son of God."

Matthew 14:22-33 *NIV*

I don't know about you, but I've never seen a water lesson where someone walked on water. Literally walked on water! Can you imagine what the disciples must have been thinking? Can you imagine being Peter walking on the stormy waves? It was only a short time that he walked on water, but it was longer than you or I.

But there you see it again. When Peter focused on the facts, the wind and the waves, he began to sink. It was Jesus, the One who is Peace and the One who is Truth, who reached out and grabbed him, saving Peter's life.

Do you not find this fascinating?! I do. I love these two

accounts. I love how many things are at play and how many aspects we learn about our Lord and our own humanity. Jesus knew both times that the storm was coming. He knew both times that the human reaction would be one of fear. Yet, he sent them anyway. He sent them directly into the storm. Although He sent them into the darkness, He went with them. He was there with them.

He is there with you and me always. He is here right now. He wasn't the One who created the storm, but he was the One who had the peace to calm the storm.

Jesus is the same yesterday as He is today and as He will be tomorrow. Jesus is the answer to having peace in the midst of all your storms. Peace while practicing medicine. Peace that transcends human understanding. The Prince of Peace is the only one who can keep you calm when you are experiencing everything but peace.

Code Stroke

I still remember the day I got that dreaded phone call. The one that no small-town emergency medicine physician wants to get in their hometown. I was sitting at the provider desk in the ED when I saw my cell light up. I saw my dad was on the caller ID, so I figured I should pick it up.

I heard a faint cracking in his voice as he said, *"Your brother has slurred speech and is not thinking clearly. Emily, I'm worried he's having a stroke. I'm bringing him in now."*

As quickly as I heard those words, my heart sank. My throat began to immediately tighten. The air felt sucked out of the room. I felt like I was gasping for air. My hands began to tingle. I knew I only had 10 minutes to prep. I stood straight up and told the nurse to get the critical bay cleared out and to bring the telemedicine monitor for stroke care into the room. I told them to call a stroke alert overhead.

I then shoved open the doors to the back hallway and walked quickly to the bathroom. The whole time, thinking, *"Please God, do not let me run into anyone!"*. All I could think was, *"I need to get to the closest bathroom. I need to get there now."*

As I was shutting the door, I heard the words *"Stroke alert, 5 minutes"*. I had heard that alert many times before. It sounded different today. Ominous, pressing.

As the lock on the door clicked shut, I had the first and only panic attack that I have ever had in my life. I began to hyperventilate and began having tingling in my face. All I could think of was, *"I cannot be the one to push tPA on my brother. God, I cannot be the one to make this call if things go badly. I cannot be the one to care for him. God, help me!"*

I have never to this day experienced such a strong sense flood my body. It came rapidly, and it was something I cannot fully describe. The best way I can describe it was an immediate wave of warmth that spread from my head all the way down to my feet. My breathing immediately slowed, and my heartbeat could no longer be felt in my throat. I now realized I was fully calm and ready for whatever came through those doors. God was with me. God was giving me His peace.

I washed my hands and turned out the light. It was time to walk down the hall. I knew now that God would be with me whatever lay on the other side of those doors.

I was rounding the corner when my brother arrived. There was a flurry of activity as he was placed on the monitor, and I began my exam. He was clearly having dysarthria or slurring of his words. It was gradually improving as the exam went on. Luckily, I saw no obvious facial droop, and there were no signs of airway compromise.

A fingerstick was checked and this showed his glucose level was within range. Dang. No low blood glucose. I was hoping it was a simple answer. Hypoglycemia was ruled out as a cause of the mental status changes as the stroke protocol continued.

As the orders were placed and he was wheeled down to the CT scanner, I continued to pray. I waited as he had full scans of his brain along with the vasculature in his head and neck. I quickly reviewed the images, waiting for the Radiologist's official read. I was relieved to see there was no large bleed. There were no obvious clots. Everything appeared normal.

What was going on?

I was continuing to stay calm and work through this stroke alert like I had done hundreds of times before. Staying focused. Taking one step at a time. Labs came back one at a time and were largely unremarkable. Things were not adding up. What had been the cause of his symptoms?

He had never experienced anything like this before. He was low risk for a stroke. He did have a remote history of migraine headaches previously but reportedly wasn't having much of a headache now. I was thinking maybe a complicated migraine could be the cause of his presentation but it still wasn't fully adding up. Something was not fitting. Deep down inside me, the gut feeling was kicking in. Something had me on edge. What were we missing?

Time went by, and no answers were found. I called the

hospitalist and presented the case. I knew that he was a borderline admit, as basically all the workups had been done regarding evaluation for a stroke. I just knew deep down, though, that we needed to keep looking.

The hospitalist didn't hesitate. He willingly accepted the admission. The ball was no longer in my court. Thank God I was able to send him out of my department.

The next phone call I got was in the afternoon the following day. I remember hearing the hospitalist's voice and wondering why he was calling me directly. He started off by saying he was very glad we admitted my brother. He went on and said he had found a large aortic aneurysm. What?! He said he couldn't explain it, and neither could the cardiologist, but he had a large ascending aneurysm, and he was going to be transferred for repair.

What had brought my brother into the ED that day did not line up with his presenting symptoms. The case did not make sense physically, yet God had lined things up so that He got the help that he needed. He did not have a dissection of the aorta that could have caused the symptoms. No rupture. Just an enlargement of his ascending aorta that had been caught because my brother had come in that day.

God knew the storm was coming to me that day. He knew that He was going to allow my brother to come in on my shift. But you know what, He sent His peace in the storm.

He knew my shortcomings. He knew what I could physically handle. Yet, He helped me come up higher. He showed me what it was like to rely on Him in the moment of one of my greatest fears. Where my ability to handle the stress failed, God's peace and presence stepped in.

This was only the start of my brother's journey. It was his heart that was the first to be repaired and revived. Although his health journey and hospitalizations were filled with multiple close calls, they also allowed us to witness the hand of God literally sparing his life.

It was in the dark nights of his journey that God was doing a greater work in him as well as me. I didn't realize it at the time, but being part of the team that sought to revive my brother's heart showed me one of the keys to reviving the heart of medicine.

His heart may have been the first to be revived but now the focus shifts to you and me. God has called each one of us to become beacons of hope in the stormy waters for our patients. He has called each one of us to anchor ourselves to Him so that we can be steady in the face of turbulent waters. We are called to carry God's peace in all circumstances. Even when we have no peace on our own.

Here is the truth. He has more than enough peace for each one of us. It is His peace that He leaves with us. It is His peace that He freely gives to us. But it is our job to ask Him for it. He will never force it on you.

It is our job to stay close to the Prince of Peace so that we can carry His peace into every room and situation he calls us to.

Jesus never promised us that it would be an easy journey. He never promised us that it would be smooth sailing. But He is calling you to journey to the other side with Him.

As you go, He promises that He will always be by your side no matter what may come. The Prince of Peace is with you always.

Take time today and begin to grow in His peace. Spend time with Him each and every day. Soak in His presence. Soak in His peace. You never know just when you or someone else will need His peace. You never know the hearts around you that are needing to be revived.

"The Lord himself will fight for you. Just stay calm."
Exodus 14:14 *NLT*

Uprooting Unforgiveness

"Get rid of all bitterness, rage and anger, brawling and slander, along with every form of malice. Be kind and compassionate to one another, forgiving each other, just as in Christ God forgave you."
Ephesians 4:31-32 *NIV*

There are few things more damaging to the health of your mind, body, and spirit than the root of unforgiveness. When this root is allowed to grow in the dark, untouched and continually watered, it has the power to destroy friendships, families, and organizations. To even destroy, on a much larger scale, towns, states, and countries.

This root is especially damaging in the field of healthcare. In a space that is supposed to bring about health and healing.

In Proverbs 4:23, it says to *"Guard your heart above all else, for it determines the course of your life."* *NLT*

This is absolutely true. When unforgiveness is not

resolved, it pollutes your heart. It is one of the strongest spiritual heart attacks there is. It impacts every area of your life. It impacts your health. It is a poison that slowly causes death.

Likewise, it impacts every area of the lives of your patients.

When God began really working in my own heart, the first root He started with was one of unforgiveness. Let me tell you, it was a rough root to pull... As I've talked with many others who are on this same path, they have said this was the first root God started working on them with as well.

Personally, I was quite offended when the subject was originally brought up. No one likes to hear that they have areas they need to fix. No one likes to have the spotlight shining on the dark areas of their life. Me? Seriously?! Not me, God. I truly believed I was NOT the one with the issue. They are the problem!! Luckily for me, God was not persuaded by my defense statement.

He did not give up on this issue with me. He continued to chip away at it, a little bit at a time. Chipping away at the icy exterior of my heart until it could be allowed to beat again. He had to heal the scars to restore the function. Of course, God had quite a few layers to peel back with me before He helped me realize that holding onto unforgiveness was destroying my heart. It was destroying my health. It was destroying the health of my closest relationships.

Perhaps you have not struggled with unforgiveness, but perhaps you know someone who has dealt with it. Or perhaps you have taken care of a patient who is bitter and angry at the world. Where you see or experience bitterness, there is always unforgiveness lurking in the shadows.

Did you take the time to wonder what their story was? What originally broke them? How did that pain start? Well, it started with a wound that was never healed. It started with an area of hurt that was kept in the dark. A root of unforgiveness that continued to fester until it turned into a stronghold of the mind.

The enemy has long been using this trick to stop God's movement in your life. To stop you from enjoying a life that is free of unforgiveness, bitterness, and anger.

Now, take a deep breath before reading the next statement. Here's another thought that may make you upset. However, it needs to be said. Did you realize that you aren't actually mad at the person who hurt you? Yes. I said that correctly. You aren't mad at that person. You are mad at the spirit behind that person. The spirit that tempted them into doing that atrocious deed.

I know. It's a tough pill to swallow when you first hear that statement, but it's time to see the truth. That person who hurt you is just a pawn. They are just a human that the enemy is working through to hurt you. To cause chaos. To create brokenness. To stir up anger. He is using them to keep you involved in a conflict so that you miss out on the things God is truly calling you to.

How can I say this? Because it is the truth. You were hurt in the physical realm, but there is so much more going on behind the scenes than you realize. The enemy is very clever. He never comes right out in plain sight. He works in the shadows. He is the darkness that is always lurking around the corner.

If you miss this truth that it is not truly the person you are battling but the forces of the spiritual realm, it will seem impossible to forgive. I am not just saying this statement without any substantive support. It is very clearly stated in the Word,

"For our struggle is not against flesh and blood, but against the rulers, against the authorities, against the powers of this dark world and against the spiritual forces of evil in the heavenly realms."
Ephesians 6:12 *NIV*

Take a moment to let that sink in. That person who hurt you was not the one who truly hurt you. That person who broke your heart, stole something from you, took your innocence, etc. That person was being controlled by another spirit.

Does this mean that person is fully bad? That they are totally evil? No. It means they are human. It means that they are like you and I, falling short of perfection.

It means that in that moment or in that period of their life, they were listening more to the lies and temptations of the enemy of their soul than to the life-giving Holy Spirit.

No matter how terrible that person seems or how shockingly terrible their act was, they are still a child of God. They are still a person that Jesus died for. So, as difficult as it is to begin looking at things that way, it is the key to being able to forgive. It is the key that unlocks your prison of offense. It is the key that allows you to take your hands off the prison bars and walk right out of the snare of the enemy.

Once you know that the being who truly harmed you was the enemy of your soul working through that person, it allows you to separate them from that action. It allows you to see them through new eyes. It allows you to see them through God's eyes.

You see, like you and I, they messed up. They missed the mark. They may have intentionally harmed you or are continuing to harm you. That is where this truth becomes even more powerful.

I am not saying to stay in a harmful situation. Hear me. That is absolutely not what I am saying. If you are in an abusive situation or one where you are in harm's way, absolutely seek help and leave the situation. That's beyond the scope of this book, though. I am saying that the more you realize that they are being used by the enemy, the more powerful your response is in choosing to forgive. In choosing the opposite of what the world tells you to do.

The world and the spirit that controls the world will tell you to get even. To fight back. To make them hurt as much as they hurt you. But you don't realize that it is just taking you down their path. A path that is taking you away from healing. Away from restoration. Away from peace. It is taking you down the same path that the enemy is hoping he can lead you down to destruction.

This is not something that just happens to one person. It happens to all of us, all of the time. The enemy is continuously stirring up division and strife. He is creating countless opportunities for offense.

This topic is never as important as it is today. All around us, we are witnessing the roots of unforgiveness turn into hotspots of rage. Of division. Of nastiness.

The Pandemic was a worldwide example of division playing out in patients' lives, in the lives of healthcare workers, in the workplace, in cities, and in government, etc. What was the division based on? It was based on a difference of opinions. The enemy incited drama that has continued to cause a divide in this nation as well as the hearts of people.

Yes, there were wrongs. Yes, it was not right. Yes, both sides believed they were right. And yes, many are still struggling with forgiveness. Struggling with the wounds that occurred. Let me ask you some tough questions, though. What is unforgiveness doing for you? Has it helped you? Do you feel justified in staying in unforgiveness? Is it helping you in any way? Is it helping your blood pressure or your tension headaches? Is it helping you to see your family in a loving manner? Is it helping you to be a good employee at work? Is it helping you to see your patients in a new light? In a way that helps you to understand where they are coming from?

Okay. Good to know.

The unforgiveness may feel good. You may feel justified. You may feel you do not have a problem, that they are the true problem. So did I. Well, we are both wrong in this case.

It's time to wake up and walk out of this prison. Forgiveness is the only way to true health and restoration. It is the only way to truly move past the hurt.

I have heard the quote, *"Not forgiving someone is like drinking poison and hoping it kills the other person."* That is exactly what you are doing when you are holding onto unforgiveness. You may be in the right. They really may have been the ones to wrong you. It is not okay, and you do not have to agree that it was okay. That is not what this is about. Forgiveness is a choice. It is what God asks us to do. It is what our Creator knows is best for us.

You may be wondering how it is possible to forgive the

person who harmed you. The spouse who cheated on you and left. The crook that took your money. The drunk driver who took the life of your family member. Here's the thing. You do not have the power to forgive. But you know the One who does.

It is only by the Holy Spirit that you can truly forgive. It is by the Spirit of God that you can be given the power to submit the offense to the only One who can truly heal the wound.

There is a reason Proverbs 20:22 (*ESV*) says, "*Do not say, "I will repay evil"; "wait for the Lord, and he will deliver you."*

You do not have the power to change the other person. You do not have the power to make the wrongs right. He does. God is the answer to unforgiveness. He is the answer you need to restore your heart. He is the answer to reviving the heart of medicine.

Only through releasing unforgiveness can you be an effective leader. An effective worker. An effective spouse. An effective human in an environment where we are continually surrounded by opportunities for offense.

I will tell you it is not an easy path, though. The path is not a wide one that you can walk on. There are many who will not want to join you when you decide to walk this way. Their eyes remain focused on the pain, not on God's promises. By doing this, their healing is blocked at the place of their deepest wounds.

The Well

This is something that my staff and I discuss frequently

at The Well, our Christian integrative wellness center in northern California. The more we reflect, the more we realize that our group was brought together during a time of division in healthcare. We were brought together in a time when we were indignant with the wrongs that we were seeing.

We were in a dark place when our doors first opened. We thought we were doing everything we could to help patients, yet we didn't realize WE needed to release the unforgiveness if we were going to help our patients find healing. We were going to have to be the change we wanted to see in healthcare.

The Well was meant to be a soft place for our patients to land. A place where providers were called to listen to our patients. Yet, we were not there to encourage them to stay in their place of bitterness. Their place of anger. No. We were there to walk the path with them and lead them to the One who could fix them.

We were called to forgive colleagues who had slandered our names. We were being asked to forgive those who had harmed others. We were called to love our Judas.

So, let me gently nudge you. You are being called to do the same right now. You are called to forgive those who have harmed you. You are called to see them in a new light. You are called to turn to the only One who has the power to help you heal from those deep wounds.

You are there to help your patients see this truth as well. You are there to open their eyes to how unforgiveness is poisoning their own health. This is not something that you will battle with one time. It is something that is continually walked out. I promise you, though, that if you take the time and turn your wounds over to the only One who has the power to heal them, it will be worth it. Not only will it bring you peace but it will be one of the most freeing things you have done in your entire life.

Take time to get quiet. Ask God to reveal areas where you are holding onto unforgiveness. Ask Him to bring to your mind the people who you have held captive by your unforgiveness. This is not just a simple request. This is necessary for your good.

"For if you forgive other people when they sin against you, your heavenly Father will also forgive you.
But if you do not forgive others their sins, your Father will not forgive your sins."
Matthew 6:14-15 *NIV*

We cannot hold onto the poison of the enemy's darts. Turn it over to God. He has the power to fight for you and to redeem even the worst situations. Release the hurt. Drain the poison. Refuse to settle in the valley of dry bones.

By choosing to forgive in a society that lives constantly offended, you will become a light that penetrates the darkness. You will be one who heals, not just gives superficial remedies that only mask the symptoms. Choosing forgiveness is a key to reviving your own heart. It is a key to reviving the heart of medicine.

THE POISON OF PRIDE

"When pride comes, then comes disgrace, but with humility comes wisdom."
Proverbs 11:2 *NIV*

Pride is literally killing patients. It is lethal to the medical industry. It is one of the largest roots that needs to be removed to revive the heart of medicine.

Are you offended by this? That is pride you are feeling. Being offended means you value yourself much more than the person who has a different opinion than you hold. You believe they cannot possibly be right. That is pride.

Pride is one of the most dangerous traits a healthcare professional can have. It is one of the biggest spiritual roots that prevents a person from seeing themselves as they truly are. It prevents one from having the ability to change. You cannot uproot what you don't realize you need to remove.

I am not talking about appropriate confidence. As a

healthcare practitioner, we should be confident in our realm. Pride is different from confidence. Pride says you believe you know everything. You constantly believe that you could not possibly be wrong.

Pride harms patients and healthcare professionals and contributes to the broken system. Pride hardens your heart. Pride is currently killing the medical industry. It is killing patients.

Why is pride so dangerous? Because it causes blindness. It causes such profound blindness that you don't even realize that you need help. How can you change what you are doing if you believe so highly in your skills that you don't think that you could improve?

Pride is behind the belittling comments that practitioners make to one another, whether out in the open or to others. Ones they put on their charts that they don't think that their patients or other practitioners will see. Or perhaps they are so prideful they don't care if they see.

Pride is the reason many patients are gaslit and told that they don't really know what is going on with their bodies. They are told that the medical professional knows much more than they do, and the patient could not possibly be right. Here is a fact. Sometimes, the practitioner is correct, but many times, the patient is.

Believing that you are infallible is the greatest delusion one could have. It is important to expose this lie if we are to begin to transform the field of medicine.

There is a reason that the scriptures say that God hates pride. There are numerous examples throughout scripture showing where pride caused the downfall of the person. Pride is the reason that Lucifer fell from heaven. It is the spiritual root of why he esteemed himself so highly that he believed that the angels should worship him like they worshipped the Lord. Pride is what turned Lucifer into Satan.

Pride is what made Eve bite into the forbidden fruit. Through deception, she believed she should have the same knowledge as God. Her pride is what started the deadly trend in humans. Her mistake is referenced in the warning, *"Pride comes before a fall."*

Pride was the reason that the tower of Babel was dismantled and the nations were scattered. It led to the downfall of Israel's first king, Saul. In his pride, he decided to disregard God's command and instead take the spoils of war which were not his to take. Pride lost him his kingship and his life.

Samson was so prideful of his strength he told a woman his secret to his strength. He was certain that he had killed thousands before and certain his strength would remain. That was until the strongest man in Israel's history lost his strength, followed by his eyesight. His fall led to him becoming the center of ridicule to all of his enemies. Pride cost him more than just his vision. It cost him his life.

Pride was the reason that Naaman was hung on the gallows. His disdain for Mordecai was so great, his pride in himself so unchecked, that his evil schemes were turned around and fell upon him.

Pharaoh's heart was hardened with pride. It was so full of this that it cost him his firstborn son, along with everyone else's firstborns in the land. It then cost him his army as they drowned in the Red Sea while chasing after the Israelites.

There are so many other examples in the scriptures that show the devastating effects of pride. They are not just meant to be stories that are read and forgotten. No, they are blueprints. They show us what not to do.

Pride blinds and pride kills. Sometimes the consequences are swift, other times there is a delay. The destination, though, is the same. We must realize the truth about pride if we are to open our eyes to the solution and avoid this trap of the enemy.

Eyes to See

Now that we see it is an issue that must be addressed, what is the solution to fixing pride? It is a change in vision. A change in perspective.

Many times, it takes a practitioner to become a patient before they begin to see their own pride. It often is a practitioner who is used to being in control, used to calling the shots, and then they are laid up in the hospital gown. A change in roles is a quick initial remedy when it comes to pride.

But does it really take this? The answer to this question is no. At least not in every case. Hopefully, a practitioner or healthcare professional will wake up before they get to this position. What they truly need, though, is a renewing of the mind. Of taking on the mind of Christ. Of being humble in spirit as the Son of God was.

Jesus was so humble that He chose to lower himself from His heavenly position. He chose to leave His divine birthright and come to Earth as a human to die for those who hated Him. To die for those whom He loved before they ever loved Him. To die for all of us sinners. You and I.

God had the hard part. He gave us the greatest example of what a lack of pride looks like. The Lord of the universe was so humble that He would choose to die for those who have no right to be prideful, yet who are.

We are asked to do nothing of this sort, but we are daily asked to lay down our pride. To daily walk with God and seek His ways. To daily look to Him as our strength and as our wisdom.

We must always seek after what He wants. What He desires for us. His will, not ours.

To let go of pride, we are going to have to be okay with our plans being disrupted. To be willing for God's plan to be our plan. We must realize we can do nothing apart from Him.

I promise you. God will reveal pride in your heart if you let Him.

The Tables Turned

I still remember when He began working on my pride. It was when He called me out of the Emergency Department. It was during the Pandemic. He began speaking to me, and I began to realize that I was going to be transitioning into a new season.

I had no clue what that season would look like. Now that I am in it, I know it was God's mercy that I didn't see the steps needed to lead me out of my position.

Of all the things I would need to lay down to follow God's call on my life, pride was a big one. One of the main hidden roots in me was pride.

One of the first steps He started me on was one of further education. Education in humility. I realized I did not know everything. Yes, a tough pill to swallow.

I still remember my uncle telling me about the Integrative Medicine program through the University of Arizona. A type of medicine that merges all the best aspects of various types of medicine. A medicine where the provider and patient partner together on their health journey. I didn't even realize that was possible in medicine. My interest was piqued.

During the pandemic, I had already had my eyes opened that Western or allopathic medicine did not hold all the answers for my patients. I just had no clue how much I didn't fully know. I didn't realize it would take continual learning every single day to be able to truly help patients.

With each passing month, though, He began taking me down this path toward a new career. He began revealing my new life and assignment for Him.

I did not forget about my emergency medicine skills and was thankful for them, but I could feel that chapter closing. I knew God was doing a new thing in my life.

I still remember being the director of the Emergency Department and knowing I had an amazing position, an amazing opportunity, but it was as if the anointing had lifted. I was no longer settled in the place I had grown accustomed to, comfortable with. I knew I could not move forward in what God had called me to by being unwilling to step out of my comfort zone.

That's the thing. You can never hold onto the old wineskins. If you are going to follow where He calls you, He is going to ask you to change. He is going to ask you to trust Him in the new.

When an opportunity opened to work at a nearby clinic, I was beyond excited. Outwardly, it seemed to align with my perfect job description. Looking back on it now, there were definitely red flags. I was so excited, though, to be moving forward on this path that I believed I should step forward in it. I thought it would be a great learning opportunity and a perfect fit.

That's the thing with red flags. They are often present in opportunities that are "good opportunities," but then later, you realize it was not a *"God opportunity"*. There is a key difference. With God opportunities, the blessing is apparent, and there is an anointing to deal with the difficulties that arise. With good opportunities, the risk v. benefit ratio is not in your favor. You do not have the grace to handle what comes your way. I learned the hard way about this crucial difference.

It was during this period that I was closing out my time in the Emergency Department and stepping into this other opportunity that I was opening up my practice called The Well. I was opening up the God opportunity that I had co-founded: a Christian integrative wellness center.

It was my goal to work at the other clinic while we were slowly building our practice in my hometown. I truly thought I was being careful. I thought I was planning ahead and being careful with my financial planning and steps forward. That was until my eyes were opened.

I still remember being at a residency week for my fellowship program in Tucson, Arizona, when God began speaking to me. It was during my time in prayer that I heard Him begin speaking about the need to be praying about the clinic I had joined. The one that seemed to offer such a shiny, red apple. One that outwardly appeared to be a fabulous opportunity. One that I was just certain was a perfect fit.

The problem was that I was blinded. Blinded by pride. Blinded by the comfort of a consistent paycheck. Blinded by outer appearance. I had been seeing through worldly vision while missing God's vision. Looking back on it now, I realize it was pride. I knew God had called me to open The Well, but I did not want to trust in only the provision of The Well. I wanted to make a way for myself.

How many times do we do that? How many times do we lack faith for the very thing that He calls us to? How do we believe we know more than the One who created us? That's simple. Pride.

A Shift is Coming

Well, it was during my trip to Tucson that I began praying and feeling very unsettled in my spirit about the clinic. The Holy Spirit was getting my attention and telling me ahead of time that another change was coming.

I knew by now that I was about to have my eyes opened again. My friend, the Holy Spirit, was warning me about the undercurrents that were present and alerting me to the danger up ahead. I will not go into the details of what happened, but I can tell you that the Holy Spirit had warned me for a reason.

It was a very short time after that I extracted myself from the other clinic, and I found myself only working at The Well. I went from having three jobs, one as a director and attending in an emergency department, to being an employee in another clinic and owning The Well, to all of a sudden, only owning The Well.

On one hand, it was much easier on my schedule. It greatly simplified my daily life; however, it was terrible for my finances. It was a cliff that my finances had catapulted off. It felt like there was no end to this free fall that I was in. Well, that was the beginning of learning humility.

To avoid total financial calamity, I immediately went back to see if I could pick up more shifts in the Emergency Department where I had worked the past 7 years. Thankfully, the same group was still running the department at that time. They welcomed me back and gave me many shifts to help me get by over those next few months. Unfortunately, they said there was also change coming for them.

They had been replaced by another group that would begin staffing the department. That group had already set up who was going to be staffing their department, and I was not one that would be included. I was told that I had *"made my choice"* by leaving the department originally and that I may be able to pick up a shift every now and again, but the shifts had been filled by other doctors. That was understandable. It hurt, but it was understandable.

It was a solid door that once again was closed right in my face. I had gone from being the director of the department to no longer being in the department in the span of 6 months' time. Something I honestly was shocked to experience.

That is the thing, though, with life, we never know what is right around the corner. Looking back now, it was a door that needed to close. I needed to be abruptly catapulted into God's full plan.

What would I have missed if I would have settled for comfort? For mediocrity? I don't know if I would have truly had the courage to fully step out into this chapter if I had not been forced to walk through my next door. I had to be broken out of what I had envisioned for my life to walk into what He wanted to do next.

That's the thing with God's next in our lives. Seasons of change are often abrupt and frequently not anticipated. That does not mean they are bad. It just means we need to up-level our faith walk. There is a reason God does not give us all the details. It would be difficult to comprehend what He is always doing.

With two doors closed in rapid succession, I realized that I was supposed to do the thing God had called me to do the entire time. The only choice now ahead of me was the God option.

The New Chapter

I realized He was asking me to stop focusing on the old. He was calling me to step into the new. To focus on growing His vision and expanding our Christian integrative wellness center, The Well. A place where the focus was on true healing: mind, body and spirit. A place where the practitioners and staff were focused on loving others more than loving ourselves. Where the focus was not on symptom management but on true healing.

Looking back now, it was over the past two years when I was stripped of financial security that was the key to laying down pride. The changes were so drastic in salary that the season included putting our property, which had been in our family's name for 40 years, on the market. I had to have a realtor come take pictures of our house, expose our private struggle with our finances and bring it out into the open.

In putting our house on the market, taking a massive pay cut, and experiencing a drastic lifestyle change to what I had grown accustomed to, God was asking me to submit my pride. To trust Him when I did not know what He was doing.

I heard the murmurings from people who were questioning and mocking this turn of events for me and my family. Gossiping about certain rooms in my house. People who thought they knew the picture of my life yet had missed the whole point.

Here's the key. I realized that God would even use this dark part of my story for His glory. I knew Him to be faithful. I knew that only He could take the parts of my story that are the most hurtful and bring blessing out of them.

This is why the Psalmist says,

"You prepare a table before me in the presence of my enemies. You anoint my head with oil; my cup overflows."
Psalm 23:5 *NIV*

God does not remove the enemies or those who openly mock you from your life, but He does allow them to be there to watch you when you succeed. When He turns things around for you.

I realized during this season that He was asking me to place everything on the altar to Him. He was asking me to trust Him and His plan, not to trust what I thought should happen. He was asking for me to lay down the fear of man. He was asking me to fully surrender everything of who I am, what I thought my life would look like, along with my hopes and dreams. He was asking if I would surrender fully to the call He had on my life.

He was asking for my *"yes"* before I knew the full details. He was inviting me to take each step forward and trust in Him every single day. To look to Him, not to money for my comfort. To look to Him, not status for my ego. To lay down the idols of my heart.

Turned Tables

How about you? Does this scare you? Have you asked God to search your own heart? Have you asked for Him to show you the way He wants your life to go? It is scary, but I can tell you that it is worth it.

Your possessions and your thoughts about how life should go cannot be taken with you to Heaven. Only your relationship with Him truly matters. Know this. When God allows these roots to be exposed, He is always doing it for your own good. He is only asking you to hand over your fake pearls to Him so He can be the one to give you back the true treasure. A treasure that cannot be bought. The treasure you will receive is an authentic and surrendered relationship with Jesus Christ. A faith that is unshakeable.

Pride is never worth it. It is never the answer. Pride corrupts. It clouds your vision. It hardens your heart. It focuses your strength only on you. It blinds you to the realization that His love is the only thing that matters.

So, today, I would encourage you to begin to talk to God about pride. Begin to ask Him to show you what's truly in your heart. Begin to ask Him to give you a new heart. One that is softened by humility. One that loves others more than yourself. A heart that has you seek His Kingdom before you seek anything else. One that helps you realize the need to come up higher and see things from His perspective. To truly understand that provision comes only from Him.

You are not in control. You must surrender control to Him. The sooner you realize that you do not hold all the answers and that He does, the sooner He will be able to use you.

I challenge you today to stop asking yourself why you are not seeing God move in your life. Stop asking God to use you, and instead, pray the following prayer. *"Lord, make me usable."* Pray this prayer and watch and see what He does. Watch to see what He reveals. Watch Him move.

Take the time today to lay down your will and your pride and watch Him revive your heart for Him. You can't step forward into all that He is calling you into if you continue to cling to the false comforts. You must have open hands so He can hand you the keys to your destiny.

More Valuable than Gold

"In a large house there are articles not only of gold and silver, but also of wood and clay; some are for special purposes and some for common use. Those who cleanse themselves from the latter will be instruments for special purposes, made holy, useful to the Master and prepared to do any good work."
2 Timothy 2:20-21 *NIV*

Close your eyes and imagine a beautiful vase filled with water. One that is very tall and multifaceted, reflecting light from multiple angles. A vase that is sitting on a countertop. It is half full of cyrstal clear, refreshing water.

Now imagine this same vase is now being filled up with even more water. The water just keeps flowing. This vase continues to be filled with water up to the very brim. You see it continuing to be filled until it is now overflowing, with water spilling out all over the counter. It runs down the countertops and even overflows onto the floor beneath it.

What started out as a simple vase filled with water has now changed the environment in which it sits.

Some would look at this and perhaps think that it looks like a mess. Some may say that you should have been more careful filling the vase so its contents didn't go outside its boundaries. I'm here to tell you, though, that you are that vase.

You are called to be a vessel that is so overflowing that you can't help but transform the environment around you. What is in you must be so powerful, so refreshing, so transforming that others can't help but be affected when you walk in the room. It is not about the package, it is all about the contents. You are to host something that is much more powerful than you can even imagine.

If you are the vase, then what is the water? What are you to be overflowing with that has the power to transform others? We will get to that in a minute.

The Midas Touch

Have you ever met a person who is talented at multiple things? Someone who is gifted in many areas? These are people who aren't just satisfied to learn one skill. No, they are always growing. Always seeking to learn more things that could be of use to them and those around them. These people are multifaceted like that vase. These are people who seem to have the Midas touch.

If you take the time to watch them closely, you will notice that whatever they do seems to succeed. Whatever they put their mind to seems to come to fruition. What they touch becomes a golden opportunity. It may not happen at first but keep watching. It may take them a few tries but you must know they are ones who will not accept defeat. They will keep pressing on toward whatever goal has been placed in front of them.

I have known various people like this over the years. Ones that I have greatly admired. Ones that seemed to host something that was supernatural. These are people who are overflowing with something that cannot be contained. It refuses to be held back.

Well, what you and I were witnessing was someone who had a spirit of excellence. They were not only hard workers, but they prospered wherever they were planted. They had wisdom in many areas. They seemed to always be over-flowing with gifts and talents.

What was it that gave them this unique edge? What made them excellent in all they set their mind to? It was a spirit of excellence. It was a spirit of wisdom. It was Living Water.

Becoming Excellent

One of the keys to reviving the heart of medicine is saturating the workers with the same spirit of wisdom as these people who are gifted in multiple areas. To instill in them a spirit of excellence. Helping them learn how to be filled with Living Water. This sounds like a large task, but it is necessary. It can be done, but we aren't the ones who can do it for them.

Let me explain.

It is not in seeking mediocrity that we can shift the atmosphere in the current healthcare system. It is not in just *"getting by"* like others that your life will have the power to transform those around you. You cannot just show up empty to your place of work and expect to be a blessing to others. No. You must be overflowing like that vase.

You must be so full that you can't help but be a blessing to others. It is by standing out that you transform your environment. By being excellent in all that you do. This is what allows you to change lives. Carrying supernatural wisdom helps you not only solve the greatest challenges for your life, it allows you to be an example to others looking to make changes in their own lives. By having an innate drive to do everything to reflect God's glory, you will become a chain breaker.

Yet, it is not in your own strength that you can do these things. You must be filled with His love that overflows out of a transformed heart.

You may be wondering; how do we do this? How do we help others grow in wisdom? How do we grow in a spirit of excellence? How do we help people truly love the patients they care for and the colleagues they work with? How can we make an impact in the lives of our friends, our family and anyone who comes across our path?

Those aren't the real questions that you are seeking though. We must ask the right questions if we are going to get to the heart of the matter.

What we need to be asking is, *"Who is behind this excellence? Who is behind wisdom? Who is behind a changed heart?"*. We find the answer to this in the book of Daniel. It is said about Daniel and his three friends:

"To these four young men God gave knowledge and

understanding of ALL kinds of literature and learning. And Daniel could understand visions and dreams of ALL kinds."
Daniel 1:7 *NIV*

It is said that Daniel especially stood out due to the excellent spirit within him. He was not just another ordinary worker or an ordinary man. His excellence is what distinguished him.

"Then this Daniel became distinguished above all the other high officials and satraps, because an excellent spirit was in him."
Daniel 6:3 *NIV*

You may be wondering why Daniel was so excellent. Why was he found to be regarded with such high esteem by those who were near him? What made him stand out? One of the kings whom Daniel served directly, answers this question for us with the following statement.

"The king asks Daniel, "I've heard about you—that you're full of the Holy Spirit, that you are very wise and have knowledge and extraordinary understanding..."
Daniel 5:14 *NIV*

The answer to the question then is very simple. The key to being excellent and to having unusual wisdom is being filled with the Holy Spirit. The key to being able to love the unlovable is having the Spirit of Christ. The key to transforming others is being filled to the brim with Living Water.

Running over. Transforming everything and everyone in our path.

Unfortunately, there are many people who do not even know what this means. Many are even fearful of the Holy Spirit. Some will stop listening when you talk about God. Even more will walk away when you talk about Jesus. But watchout when you bring up the Holy Spirit! You never know what buttons will be pushed.

Many people have head knowledge and a basic understanding of Jesus. They realize He is the part of the Godhead that became flesh. They understand that Jesus clothed himself in humanity to walk this Earth and to die for beings that He created. They witnessed His life as the epitome of Heaven touching Earth.

Many understand about God the Father. Some who have unfortunately been brought up in a legalistic and religious environment have been conditioned to be fearful of the Father. Others, however, have made it a focus to lean into the Father. They connect the truth that Jesus is a reflection of who the Father is and that He carried out exactly what the Father told him to do. They then understand that the Father is loving. They realize Jesus carries the heart of the Father and that God the Father is trustworthy and loving.

When it comes to the Holy Spirit, though, many have been especially confused. They don't know what to think of this mysterious part of God. Even worse than not knowing, many have fallen for the lies of the enemy. Many have been blinded. They have listened to lies that make us afraid of our greatest gift. Of our Advocate. Our Ally. The part of the Godhead that was sent to transform our hearts and lives.

If you take time to think about it, it is actually quite

clever how the enemy has waged a war against the Holy Spirit. How he has created such division even in Christianity about one of the members of the Trinity. The one whom Jesus told us about who would be a special blessing for us after He returned to Heaven.

The Holy Spirit is the portion of the Trinity that was mentioned over 260 times in the New Testament alone. One who has been referred to by various names which portray portions of identity: The Spirit of God, the Spirit of Christ, the eternal Spirit, the Spirit of truth, the Spirit of grace, the Spirit of glory, the Spirit of life, the Spirit of wisdom and revelation, the Comforter, the Spirit of promise, the Spirit of adoption, the Spirit of holiness, the Spirit of faith. Helper. Advocate. Friend. Prince of Peace.

He has been represented by 6 different emblems that show His nature and mission: the Dove, Water, Oil, a Seal, Wind and Fire. By just reading these different names and different representations of the Holy Spirit, one can't overlook how clearly the Word of God has spoken about such an important piece of the Trinity. Yet, some pastors today still preach a message that completely disregards the Holy Spirit. When they do this, they are unknowingly preaching a powerless message.

Likewise, in medicine, those who are caring for patients without the close connection to the Holy Spirit are missing the key difference between being a clinician versus being a healer. They have eyes but do not see. They have ears but do not hear. They are empty vessels that are lacking Living Water and lacking the power to transform others.

Some have been misled by the lie that the Holy Spirit and the gifts of the Holy Spirit are no longer available. Some believe that the Holy Spirit was only poured out on the day of Pentecost and that He is not still active in us today. Others have been taught that only "*weird*" Christians are filled with the Holy Spirit.

Why does this line of thought seem eerily familiar to a grade school mentality? Why does this reasoning seem prevalent in a society blinded by conformity today? Because the enemy tries to use cancel culture in the church to cancel our greatest gift and Advocate while we are on this Earth. He uses the tactics of the world against those who are not supposed to be conforming to the world.

Unfortunately, this is not the first time that the enemy has preached from a pulpit. He knew he couldn't kill the church through martyrdom, so he decided to join the church and pervert its messages. We are seeing this become more common with each passing day. Churches that water down the truth just enough to be accepted and palatable to the world around them. Messages that seem pleasant to the ears, yet when held to the standards of the Word, completely miss the whole point.

Half truths are just full lies dressed up and given another name.

The Holy Spirit was left for us to be our guide. To live in us as the Spirit of Christ. To guide us in our daily walk with Him. To guide us in all our decisions. It is the Holy Spirit that connects us to the mind of Christ and who fills us with Living Water.

Those who have received the Holy Spirit are transformed. Those who are daily connected with Him are overflowing with His presence and with His love. They cannot help but be transformed by the love of One who is love.

If you still are hesitant about the Holy Spirit, don't just take my word on it. Listen to the words of your Creator. Jesus himself spoke directly about sending us the Holy Spirit. He said that it would be an advantage for us when He came. Our Savior was making sure we were aware of the Gift of His Presence that would be with us for all time.

"But I tell you the truth, it is to your advantage that I go away; for if I do not go away, the Helper (Comforter, Advocate, Intercessor—Counselor, Strengthener, Standby) will not come to you; but if I go, I will send Him (the Holy Spirit) to you".
John 16:7 AMP

If Jesus spoke so highly of the Holy Spirit, then it would seem highly beneficial for us to take notice. It is to our greatest good that we learn who the Holy Spirit is and actively seek to be filled with the Holy Spirit. Why would we want to miss out on such an important person of God?

"But the Advocate, the Holy Spirit, whom the Father will send in my name, will teach you all things and will remind you of everything I have said to you."
John 14:26 *NIV*

Paul, arguably the greatest apostle and teacher of all time, knew the importance of the Holy Spirit. The person who wrote at least 25% of the New Testament was very specific about speaking of the need to receive the Holy Spirit.

"While Apollos was at Corinth, Paul took the road through the

interior and arrived at Ephesus. There he found some disciplesand asked them, "Did you receive the Holy Spirit when you believed?"
They answered, "No, we have not even heard that there is a Holy Spirit."
So Paul asked, "Then what baptism did you receive?"
"John's baptism," they replied.
Paul said, "John's baptism was a baptism of repentance. He told the people to believe in the one coming after him, that is, in Jesus."On hearing this, they were baptized in the name of the Lord Jesus. When Paul placed his hands on them, the Holy Spirit came on them, and they spoke in tongues and prophesied"
Acts 19:1-6 *NIV*

The Holy Spirit is the piece to having a renewed mind and being born again. He is the difference between religion and relationship. He is the difference between being a health-care professional who is average and lukewarm and one who is a vessel used to heal patients in mind, body and spirit.

Jesus is the key to our salvation, and the Holy Spirit is the key to receiving a renewed mind. To receiving the mind of Christ. To living this life as an overcomer. To bringing the change that we want to see in the world. He is the connection to bringing Heaven to Earth.

Unfortunately, the enemy has lulled many people to sleep regarding this. He has caused many in the church to focus on legalism, to be deadened by the law. Yet, the law does not have the power to save because all fall short of the law.

You must realize that the law will never change one's

heart or actions. All will fall short when we are judged by the law. This is why Jesus came and fulfilled the law. This is why we are under a new covenant, one that is full of grace. One that is not based merely on our works but based on the finished work of Jesus Christ dying on the cross. It is salvation by grace through faith in our Redeemer.

The same is true in medicine. Rules and regulations will not change the heart of the practitioners. Legislation will not restore the art of medicine. It may help. It hopefully will cut some of the unnecessary red tape and block some of the corruption that is running rampant these days. Yet, it will not revive the heart of medicine.

The Holy Spirit is the key to true repentance and heart change whether it is in your work place or your home. He is the key to transforming your relationship with your spouse, your friends and your inner circle and He is the key to truly healing patients.

In contrast, religion is focused on following a set of rules. On following guidelines outside ourselves in an effort to look like we have changed. It is a superficial focus and it does not have any power to transform. Just ask the religious leaders who crucified Christ. They were the most cold-hearted vipers who were the most religious ones of their day. We aren't called to follow in their footsteps.

I am not saying that we are to throw out the law. Absolutely not. But if you are only focused on the law and trying to dictate a relationship with God without a true renewing of the mind and spirit, you will fail every time.

You do not have the power to overcome in this life when relying on your own willpower and strength. You do not have the power to effect true change in any environment you step into on your own. It is only through Jesus who sent us the Holy Spirit that we can be overcomers. It is through His Spirit that we can shift the atmosphere of our homes, our workplaces and our nation.

Relationship with God and being filled with the Holy Spirit are what transform people from the inside out. It is only by His grace that we can be born again. It is only by the power of the Holy Spirit that we can be new creations. That we can do what we, in our own power, are powerless to do.

That is why the enemy has caused such confusion when it comes to the Holy Spirit. This is why you have many that preach a powerless gospel.

Many Christians who you run into are not showing the fruit of the Holy Spirit in their lives. They are lukewarm. There are many who are set on following a list of rules or regulations but who are missing the entire point of the gospel. Ones who have warmed pews for years without allowing their hearts to be warmed or their minds to be renewed.

Jesus was clear on this when he summed up the law and the prophets. He said we are to love God first and to love our neighbor as ourselves. That is the whole point of the entire Bible. That is the whole point of a true relationship with God.

We cannot truly love others or love God without the transforming power of the Holy Spirit. We cannot overflow with the wisdom and love of God if we are devoid of the Holy Spirit.

This is not about shaming others. It is about bringing light to a subject that is necessary when working to transform medicine. It is a key piece to reviving the hearts of those who make up the field of medicine. We must be transformed from the inside out if we are truly going to be a light for others. You must be overflowing with the Holy Spirit if others are going to sense His presence and love in your life.

You are not called to be an empty Christian who just waits for God to come back and does nothing to advance His kingdom on Earth. Will you be saved? Absolutely. But you will miss the main point of what Jesus showed us while on Earth. You will miss what it means to live life as a reflection of Christ. You will blindly miss what it looks like to bring Heaven to others here on Earth.

Why would people want to become followers of Christ if they only see Christians who are upset all the time, who do not truly love others and who are focused only on what happens within the four walls of a church? Why would others want to experience what we have if they only see lack? Lack of love, lack of true repentance, lack of the fruits of the Spirit.

Medicine cannot be transformed from the outside in. It cannot be changed by creating more rules and regulations. You cannot dictate to others that they are to be kind to patients and that they are to treat them as if they were family. To treat others as they would themselves want to be treated.

How have you felt when you have been cared for by individuals who did not have a heart for others? If you haven't experienced what it is to work with others whose hearts are hardened or to be cared for by them, then I am honestly shocked. It is very jarring and unsettling. They are cold clinicians. They are not healers.

It is a heart change that must occur. The heart of medicine needs a revival. It is in need of restoration. It is a reviving of the heart of the healthcare provider that is the key to reviving the heart of medicine.

If the healthcare system was made up of individuals who were filled with the heart of God and overflowing with the Holy Spirit, there would be no other option for medicine to be transformed. There would be no other option for our patients to be changed. To experience a love that transforms their lives.

I promise you; patients can tell the difference. Colleagues can tell the difference when you are empty of His love. They can also tell a difference when your cup runneth over (or the vase, as it were).

When you are functioning from a place of hurt, from a place of a non-renewed mind, from a place that is focused on just making money and getting through your day. Others can sense that. When you are filled more with the spirit of mankind and not the Holy Spirit, you are causing harm to those who you are trying to heal. When you are caring for a person's family member and treasure, and you are treating it like an obligation and not a gift, people take notice.

Running on Empty

Many have grown cold to what they were originally called to do. They went into healthcare to help others, yet they have become burned out. They have become overwhelmed by the drain that it has created in their own life. They are running on empty and trying to heal others from a place of lack.

I am not saying this to shame them. I understand burnout. I was in this place. I can talk from a place of overcoming it. You must understand the truth, though. You cannot give away what you lack.

You cannot bring peace if you yourself do not have peace. You cannot be loving if you are not overflowing with God's love. You cannot have true wisdom and be excellent if you are not filled with the Spirit, who is excellent, who is the essence of wisdom.

So, I challenge you today. Seek after excellence. Seek after wisdom. Seek after the Holy Spirit.

To change the healthcare system, we must break out of the current model. By not seeking after superficial change but by seeking to be fully renewed with the Mind of Christ. It is by spending time in God's presence. By accepting Jesus Christ and what His gift of salvation is. By opening yourself up to the Holy Spirit that you will be transformed.

Just as we are beings who are mind, body and spirit, it is in this aspect that we are to reflect the Trinity. We are also called to reflect the heart of the Father. We cannot do this if we disregard our Helper. If we disregard the Gift who was sent as our guide on this journey.

I encourage you to take the time today to read more about the Holy Spirit. Don't just take my word on it. Search the scriptures for yourself. See that it was the Spirit who was hovering over the waters from the start of creation. Learn that He is hovering over us now. Come to know that He is always present, always hoping to be invited in.

Understand that it was the Holy Spirit that Jesus was filled with while walking here on Earth. That it was the Holy Spirit that was sent to the church to give power to the body. To those who would believe and accept Him.

It is the Holy Spirit that is the key to showing others who God truly is. It is the Holy Spirit that is the Spirit behind reviving the heart of medicine. He is needed to overflow in all areas of our lives so that we can be a blessing to everyone who comes across our path.

I challenge you to take time today to soak in His presence. Take time to learn of the mysterious one of the Godhead. Of the One who is the Spirit of wisdom, of revelation and of excellence.

Stop settling for mediocrity. Refuse to "just get by" in your walk with God or your work in the field of healthcare. There is One who is here to guide you in all decisions and in every area of life. He will reveal to you His secrets if you will only trust Him.

Surrender to the Holy Spirit. Ask Him into your heart today and watch what He will do. The Holy Spirit is a key to reviving your heart and the heart of medicine.

Supernatural Intelligence

"What we have received is not the spirit of the world, but the Spirit who is from God, so that we may understand what God has freely given us. This is what we speak, not in words taught us by human wisdom but in words taught by the Spirit, explaining spiritual realities with Spirit-taught words."
1 Corinthians 2:12-13 *NIV*

There are times in life when we make great decisions. Times where everything falls easily into place. We have done the training. We have watched the lectures. We have read the books. Times where we know the answer, we make the shot, or we get the deal. It just comes naturally.

But there are also times when we don't have the answers... at least initially. Times where we came so close to making the wrong call. Split-second decisions that could cost someone their life.

That's the thing about medicine. No one has all the answers. Patients don't always follow the book. Circumstances don't always line up. That is why they call it the practice of medicine. We don't always get it right.

Here's the key, though. Something that should give you much comfort, especially as a practitioner or as a patient. We have an advantage. Some would say an unfair advantage. We are connected to the iCloud of all iClouds. The dictionary of all dictionaries. The Up-To-Date of all Up-To-Dates.

That's right, we have access to supernatural intelligence. The whisperings of the Holy Spirit. Our advocate in practicing medicine in all situations. It is this source of divine information that can step in to save a life… just in time.

"And I say unto you, Ask, and it shall be given you; seek, and ye shall find; knock, and it shall be opened unto you. For every one that asketh receiveth; and he that seeketh findeth; and to him that knocketh it shall be opened".
Luke 11:9-10 *KJV*

Look Again

It was one of the most difficult cases in the Emergency Department that I was taking care of when I heard the phrase, "*Look again*".

It had all started out fairly benign. Just a patient being placed in a hall bed. I had seen this hundreds of times before. There was nothing really special about how they came in or what their story was. It was just another day in a small-town Emergency Department.

As I rounded the corner to receive report from the paramedic, I listened intently to the story. The person laying in the bed in front of me looked fairly young and overall didn't appear to be in bad shape. They had good color and appeared to be moving all extremities. They looked nervous, but all of us would be if we had a crowd of strangers standing over us, watching our every move. As I listened further though, an unusual story unfolded that I couldn't quite explain.

As the paramedic gave the report, they talked about the patient working outside and then suddenly reporting a numb sensation that spread over their entire body. It was a numbness that affected all limbs. It was a sensation that had never occurred before. They elucidated further saying there was a brief period of change in vision, however this had since been resolved. Only the numbness remained.

As I listened further, I began to go over the differential in my head. Stroke, anxiety, complicated migraine. Hmm, what could cause all the symptoms and bring the picture together?

The symptoms had recently started. I realized I needed to urgently find the answer. This appeared to be a simple case from the start, but I was quickly becoming aware that it wasn't that simple. The patient was placed in a hall bed, which typically meant they were not as urgent of a case, but I couldn't shake the feeling. I needed to solve this, and I needed to do it quickly.

After performing a quick exam, I went back to the provider's office and placed orders. I decided to go with a stroke alert so I could quickly get imaging going. This is when I heard, *"Stop. Look again."* It was faint at first, but then it was getting stronger. It was nothing that could be audibly heard. They were words that were placed in my spirit. Words that were authoritative, yet kind.

I was feeling more uneasy by the minute. What was I missing?

I got out of my chair again. The orders had already been placed, and the CT technician was on their way. I rounded the corner again. What was I missing? What had I overlooked?

As I got to the patient's bed, I noticed this time that the blood pressure was low. Much lower than I would expect for how they looked clinically. Much lower than I would expect for a young and healthy-appearing individual. Well, vitals are called vital for a reason. You learn this truth early on in medicine and you relearn it at various times throughout your career. Vitals tell a large portion about the patient's condition. You have to respect vitals.

I noted the low blood pressure but still didn't have the answer. What was I missing?

The CT technician began wheeling the patient to the scanner. My time to analyze was over. I knew he would be at the scanner momentarily. As I went back to my computer, the words *"Aortic Dissection"* flashed in front of my eyes. There it was, and it was in bold. Chills spread over me. My chair now felt like I was sitting on needles. I couldn't get out of it quickly enough.

An aortic dissection is a big deal. It means there is a tear in the wall of the most important vessel in your body. It means death if not dealt with.

It was no longer a hunch. No, deep down, I knew that God was speaking. He was breaking through my own weakness and was bringing His strength. His wisdom. His spiritual intelligence. In an instant, I knew I needed to change the orders.

It was not a stroke alert that was needed with a CT of the head and neck. No, it was a different imaging series I needed to focus on. A CT angiogram of the chest and abdomen.

I ran down the hallway and burst open the door to the CT technician's dark room, and he looked at me with shock and some annoyance. "*Can I help you?*" I rapidly told him I was giving him a verbal order to change the imaging. I was going to do a CT head and a CT-angiogram of the chest/abdomen/pelvis. He looked at me and told me something that gave me more chills. He said, "*Well, you better be sure. You get one shot. If I inject the dye into their system, I can either look at the vessels in the brain and neck, or I can look at the vessels in the chest and abdomen. You can't have both. It's your call, doc*".

I paused for a moment. Took a breath. Then said, "*Change it. Do the aorta protocol.*"

I went back down the hall and began praying. Praying I wasn't wrong. Praying that I hadn't cost this young patient their life by my rapid decision based on a feeling and a word I saw. Ten minutes went by before I received the call. Ten minutes that felt like hours.

On the other end of the phone was my friend, the CT technician. He sounded a bit shocked. He said, "*You were right. It's the largest aortic dissection I've ever seen. It's dissected from the root of the heart all the way to the iliac vessels. Doc, I'm not sure this one is going to make it*". My heart sank.

I was glad I had made the right call but I knew time was not in our favor. I quickly made another phone call. I called the closest facility, which was one hour away. I knew I needed a facility that had a cardiovascular surgeon and I needed this immediately.

I started with the transfer center. The lady on the phone said she was sorry, but they were totally full and not accepting any transfers at this time. I reiterated the need for an emergent transfer, and I received the same response. No, not at this time.

I began calling other facilities. I eventually reached a facility 4 hours away. I spoke to their cardiovascular surgeon. She was very sympathetic and readily agreed to accept the case. But her last words before getting off the phone were startling. She said, *"I'll be happy to take them. But he will likely die on the way. Prep the family for this"*.

I got off the phone and went back into the room to talk again with the patient and their family. There wasn't a dry eye in the place. Both the patient and their parents knew this may be it. I walked out of the room feeling sick. No. This patient wasn't going to go like this.

There was a reason that I had heard the words *"Aortic dissection"*. That was not in vain. I was not given this information if they were just going to die. I would not accept this. So, I began calling. This time, I bypassed the transfer call center. This time, I looked at another sheet and found the direct cell number of a cardiovascular surgeon at the first center.

I called him three times. The first time, I was disappointed. The second time, I got more stubborn. The third time, he picked up.

I rapidly told him the story. I told him the age of the patient, the results of the scan and that he was their only hope. That he had the skills my patient needed to save their life. He needed a miracle, and I was asking him to be part of this. It took less than a couple of minutes of convincing, but he agreed. He said he would personally call the transfer center and make a way. He said that if he had to put my patient in a hall bed on the way to the OR to get them there, he would get them to the OR.

I went back into the room, elated. The parents and the patient were shocked. They had been preparing to travel four hours and were prepared the patient was going to die. A glimmer of hope was beginning to be felt.

The EMS crew was contacted again, this time for a transfer to the closer facility. They rapidly came and packaged up the patient and their chart. They knew they were going code 3 to the next facility. Lights and sirens all the way.

I felt a sigh of relief as I saw them leave through those double doors. My patient had a fighting chance. Now we wait. It was several hours later, I got the call. I was finishing up my shift when I was notified that my patient had begun to deteriorate rapidly as he arrived at the facility. The call that said that his story came close to ending but was not over yet.

The surgeon had been true to his word. He was a rockstar. Cocky, but deservedly so. He had gotten the patient to the operating suite just in time. He had repaired the massive aortic dissection, and the patient was now in recovery. This patient had survived the unsurvivable. Their life was spared, at least for the time being.

I went home and cried that night. Cried that this had happened. Cried that things had been so close for this patient. But mostly cried out of thankfulness for the divine insight that was given in the nick of time.

I realized the blessing of having a surgeon who was skilled and willing to make the impossible happen. One who used his skills to revive another's life. A God who had come near to make up for my own inadequacies as a provider.

The patient was safe.

The recipe for his case was divine timing, supernatural intelligence and a team that was unwilling to give up. This is the combo you want when you are a patient. This is the team you need to save a life.

Why Did You Make the call?

It was a few years later, during my last month in the ED, that I saw this patient again. I had seen them a couple of years prior when they came in to thank me for being part of the team that saved their life.

This time, though, they stood before me and asked a question. This time, they were not the patient in front of me. Their significant other was. They got really quiet and then looked at me and asked, *"I've been thinking about this for the past few years. What made you make the call? What made you change the scan?"*

They went on to say that the surgeon had told them he was shocked that I had picked up the diagnosis and had changed the scan. They didn't realize how close they had truly come to having a missed diagnosis that would have cost them their life.

I got quiet and told the truth. It's not a truth that physicians like to say. I told them, *"I didn't know what was going on. I knew I was missing something."* I went on to explain that I had gone back to my desk and begun praying for wisdom. Praying for answers, and that was when I heard, *"Look again"*. I went on to tell them that it was in looking again that I saw the abnormal vital signs and then saw the phrase, *"Aortic dissection"*.

I told them that it wasn't me who made the call. It was God. They began crying as I honestly confessed this. I went on. I said what was on my heart to say to the patient in that vulnerable moment. I told them, *"There is a reason you are alive. There is a reason that you survived what should have killed you. There is a reason the events lined up to spare your life. You have a great calling on your life. It's up to you to follow it."*

I walked out of the room that day, three years later from that first visit, knowing I had seen God's hand. Knowing that this patient needed to hear this message. Knowing that it wasn't a random occurrence that they survived the unsurvivable.

SQ/IQ

Supernatural intelligence is not of New Age and is not in SciFi thrillers. No. True supernatural intelligence is the Holy Spirit's gift to all who choose to walk with Him. It is for patients and it is for providers. It is for all who seek Him.

I am not special. I am just a human who is imperfect and who needs a perfect God. So are you. I am here to tell you, though, that you want a provider who relies on supernatural intelligence. You want to be a provider who has supernatural intelligence.

You have to realize that, as a provider, you cannot

possibly know everything. You must be a provider who is keyed into the voice of the Holy Spirit. The true Advocate.

Just imagine what the practice of medicine would be like if more of us were willing to step out in this manner. To step out in faith. Asking simply for help when we don't even know the words to speak. Asking for guidance. Asking for wisdom. Asking for answers.

If you are in the practice of medicine, aka the ministry of healing, you have access to supernatural intelligence. Let this sink in. You have a high IQ if you are currently caring for patients. At least, I would hope that you have a high IQ. You must have knowledge to adequately care for a human being. With that said, you may be missing a key piece of intelligence. It is the SQ or supernatural intelligence portion that you may be missing.

Don't get me wrong. You should absolutely study. You should learn all that you can learn. You should do everything you can to excel in your field. But then you need to stop and take a deep breath. Look up. Look to the One who called you to the ministry of healing. Look to the One who knows you better than you know yourself.

You have access to the One who holds all the answers. The One who created the patient who is sitting there right in front of you. He has the answers that you seek. He has the orders you should place. He can speak to you and tell you the next steps.

So, the next time you feel weak or perplexed, the next time that you are up against a wall and don't know what to do, keep going. Do not give up. Do not stop seeking. Look to the One who knows everything and who is your ever-present help in times of trouble.

IQ is great, but SQ is even greater. Knowledge is important, but supernatural intelligence and wisdom from God trumps knowledge.

You are on a journey learning the keys you need to renew your heart and mind. You are on a journey of one of the greatest movements in medicine. A journey to revive the heart of medicine. We cannot revive our hearts or revive the heart of medicine without supernatural intelligence. We must rise higher if we are to bring others with us on this journey.

So today, look to your Maker. Look to the only One with true supernatural intelligence. Take time learning who He is. Asking Him questions.

He is a good Father. He is waiting for you to just sit at His feet and see Him through new eyes again. Stop being a Martha. Learn to be a Mary. Learn to love the One who has all power to renew your mind.

Have eyes that see. Have ears that hear. Seek after your Creator, and He will give you the keys to care for His Creation.

Supernatural intelligence is a key He will impart to you when you are close to Him. If you seek after Him with your whole heart, not the world, you will be given more than you ever thought possible. He is your Guide. He is the key to renewing your mind and reviving the heart of medicine.

Wisdom is available if you know the right place to look.

"If any of you lacks wisdom, you should ask God, who gives generously to all without finding fault, and it will be given to you."
James 1:5 *NIV*

"For wisdom will enter your heart, and knowledge will be pleasant to your soul. Discretion will protect you, and understanding will guard you."
Proverbs 2:10-11 *NIV*

"The fear of the Lord is the beginning of wisdom, and knowledge of the Holy One is understanding."
Proverbs 9:10 *NIV*

Arrest Anxiety

"Do not be anxious about anything, but in everything by prayer and supplication with thanksgiving let your requests be made known to God. And the peace of God, which surpasses all understanding, will guard your hearts and your minds in Christ Jesus."
Philippians 4: 6-7 *ESV*

You cannot transform medicine if you are unable to move through fear and anxiety. You cannot be effective in your line of work if you are paralyzed by the fear of the unknown.

Every step of training, of learning new skills, of starting a new job, of ending your current chapter and beginning another one, of meeting new people, or of treating new conditions carries with it the unknown. Uncertainty of success, uncertainty of what will come, and uncertainty of your abilities.

Here is the thing, uncertainty is a constant. You will never escape uncertainty if you are alive and breathing.

Working through uncertainty in a healthy way is a necessary part of advancing and moving forward in your line of work. But anxiety can stop that progression dead in its tracks. It can literally steal your future.

Anxiety robs today's joy by focusing on tomorrow's perceived shadows. It is simply a stronghold. You may not have thought of it in these terms, but have you ever wondered what a stronghold is? Have you wondered why this word is mentioned over 50 times in the Bible?

A stronghold is a fortified place, a refuge, or a place of defense. In the Old Testament, it was often used to describe a physical city or location. One that was very protected and difficult to infiltrate. In the New Testament, though, under the new covenant, strongholds refer to spiritual challenges that must be overcome. A place of enemy encampment in the mind regarding a certain issue.

A stronghold is a place where the enemy has confused you with so many continual lies that you have finally accepted that this is just a part of your personality. That this is just who you are. When you accept these lies, you have taken a bite of his apple. Like any issue, you must first recognize a stronghold is present before you learn how to deal with it. Anxiety is a common stronghold for many people.

So many of the things that worry us or that we focus on when our thoughts are spiraling are things that will never happen. We are literally wasting our time and mental energy on events that very likely will never come to pass.

Here is the truth. The enemy is using this tactic against you. Not only is he using it against you, but he is also using it against your family and friends. And he is using it against your patients.

Anxiety drains you of the energy you need to accomplish what is staring at you today. It robs you of something before you even have the ability to obtain it. The enemy comes to steal, kill, and destroy. We should not be shocked by this.

Don't get me wrong. It is good to be a planner. It is good to be looking ahead and preparing for your future. It is necessary to not stay stuck in the past. But being stuck on the hamster wheel of continuous thoughts running through your head of what possibly could go wrong is not an effective strategy.

Anxiety leads to turning to the wrong things… it leads to numbing behaviors such as drinking alcohol, using other drugs, over-shopping, overeating, etc. When you are racked with anxiety, you are literally looking for anything to distract your mind from the gloomy picture that is now parading through your imagination.

This may not be something you struggle with, but I would highly recommend you keep reading. You are not just learning about this for yourself or your loved ones. Your patients must also know how to fight the stronghold of anxiety.

So now that you know that anxiety is a stronghold and it is something that must be overcome in the field of healthcare for you and your patients, then what is the antidote? It is simple. It is the Truth.

The Light of Truth

Lies are always overcome by Truth. Darkness is broken by light. The enemy's encampment is exposed when his lies are replaced by the Truth.

What does this look like in real life? You are right now looking at the facts that you believe you are seeing. The amount of money in your bank account or, the giant load of debt, the never-ending to-do list or the multiple skills you are still wanting to learn. You are seeing facts. The numbers, the letters, the skills, etc. but you are not looking at the Truth.

You are not looking at the One who is the supplier of all your needs. You are not looking at the one who told you that you can do all things through Christ Jesus, who strengthens you. You are not looking at the One who said He would never leave you nor forsake you.

You are using your mind, but you are using it in the wrong manner. You are wasting its amazing abilities on basic ground level work. It is not just prayer, worship, time in church, or listening to a sermon that will change your mind. These are all good things, don't get me wrong. I want to encourage you to do these things and to do them often.

Yet, you can sit on a church pew or worship so much that you lose your voice your entire life and still be struggling with anxiety and other strongholds. You must know how to effectively deal with this. You must learn that there is a battlefield that is also in the mind. You must learn how to tear strongholds down. You must learn to effectively use mental warfare with the Truth of God's word over all circumstances that are taunting you.

The Goliaths do not just drop by wishing them away. You have to learn the weapons of warfare. You have to realize how to pull up these weeds by the root.

Paul explains this perfectly regarding the way we are to battle with anxiety and other mental strongholds.

"Finally, brothers and sisters, whatever is true, whatever is noble, whatever is right, whatever is pure, whatever is lovely, whatever is admirable—if anything is excellent or praiseworthy—think about such things."
Philippians 4:8 *NIV*

You are probably thinking about how this applies to you. I see my situation, and it is not pure or lovely. How do I use this when I am spiraling?

You take the verse and truly understand what it is saying ahead of time. You ask the Holy Spirit to give you a revelation of what it means. You keep reading the Word until it starts talking back to you. You dissect each portion of it and go to battle with the information you gained from it.

When you hear the lie that you are not enough, you replace it with the Truth:

"I praise you because I am fearfully and wonderfully made..."
Psalm 139:14 *NIV*

When you believe you are never going to recover financially or make enough to provide for your family, you replace it with the Truth:

"And my God will supply every need of yours according to his riches in glory in Christ Jesus".
Philippians 4:19 *ESV*

When you are worried that you cannot handle the pain of your current situation, you replace it with the Truth:

"And after you have suffered a little while, the God of all grace, who has called you to his eternal glory in Christ, will himself restore, confirm, strengthen, and establish you."
1 Peter 5:10 *ESV*

You have to be prepared before the fight surrounds you.. You don't just show up to a shift without doing any preparation for years ahead of time. You don't just wish to become a nurse and not do any studying or clinical time. You don't become a physician by accident. You have to strive to become great. You work hard to hold onto the responsibility that you have.

It is the same work in the spiritual realm. It is identical when learning the art of overcoming mental warfare. Of learning the art of tearing down mental strongholds.

You will not be effective by staring at your giant. You will not win the battle of the mind if you are only focused on situations that are causing you fear and anxiety. You will not simply win by repeating mantras that don't have the power of God behind them.

You must overcome by God's Truth. By being so secure in your relationship with God, you cannot be moved. By continually replacing the lies with God's truth about you and the situation that you are facing. You must constantly be battling against the lies.

I will let you in on something personal for me. This is something I go to battle with every single day. That's right. Running my own business in healthcare has been the most anxiety-provoking thing I have ever done in my entire life.

When God called me out of emergency medicine and had me step into the role of one of the founders of The Well, it was a giant I was staring down. People were watching and waiting, just seeing if we were going to sink or swim.

Every single day, I had to strengthen myself in God to take on the challenges of the day. I did not have all the skills or the resources I needed. Not by any measure.

Honestly, if things had not happened the exact way they did, I do not know if I would have had the courage on my own to take that leap. If I was not surrounded by such amazing people in my life, I would have been overcome by the lies. God knew what I could handle and what I did not have the strength to carry. He has been the constant in carrying me these first two years of our medical practice.

If I had not had a relationship with God all these years, learning how He moves, listening to how He speaks, and learning how the Word applies in my life, then I would have immediately sunk. Every day knowing that I am not only responsible for my patients, but I am leading a team of amazing staff is extremely sobering. It is always present in my mind when I wake up, throughout the day and when I go to bed at night.

I know that these women have risked it all to give patients a chance at healthcare that is not the standard. They have fought tirelessly against slander, and the Lord has turned the sting from these arrows into the most amazing grit I have ever seen. He has taken the attacks and opened our eyes to the greatest opportunities for forgiveness. He has given us examples of our battles that we can share with our patients to encourage them. He is redeeming the pain. Redeeming our stories.

Like me, though, they are fighting anxiety in themselves and their patients every single day. Doing something that is breaking out of the mold is anxiety provoking.

Running a Christian integrative wellness center, where we are going after healing on all levels, mind, body, and spirit, is not for the faint of heart. It is the single largest challenge I have ever tackled. Even harder than my 10 years in emergency medicine and going through a divorce. In the line of work we do, we are not only fighting our own battles for health, but we are battling on behalf of our patients. Working to show them love, care and respect when they have often not experienced this in many of their health journeys.

Looking to find true answers to the roots of disease in their life is not quick, and it is definitely not easy. Breaking down barriers that each person has, along with the barriers we are fighting in the current medical culture, is exhausting and overwhelming at times.

Not all who started on this journey are still with us. The path is narrow, and there are distractions and land mines always up ahead. The enemy constantly uses tactics against each one of us personally and as a group. He tries offense, manipulation and deception. Yet, light always overcomes the darkness. God never leaves us to battle alone. There is always a fourth one in the fire with us. The enemy continually sends arrows our way, but God is always protecting. He is always on the move and guiding us. He is always lifting us up.

In the last two years, I have seen God's hand move in the most amazing of ways. In witnessing what I have, I have gone deeper from head knowledge of God into heart knowledge of Him.

The fires have burned off the impurities. They have refocused our vision.

I have also witnessed patients view God in a whole new light. I have seen lives transformed. I have seen healing on all levels. Though there have been great challenges, I have had the blessing to be part of an amazing group of women that has been forged in the fires of the pandemic and came out warriors for God and for their fellow man.

So, the battles of the mind are not going to overcome our mission. The stronghold of anxiety will bow to God's word. The mission that we have been called to is much greater than these momentary struggles. We are to be stewards of this movement. It is not ours, it is His.

Likewise, you are called to be a chain breaker. You are called to not only fight these battles for yourself but for others. You must not give in to the enemy.

Once you learn these tactics, you are then able to teach others. Just like in medicine, the saying is, *"You see one, you do one, then you teach one."* The same is true with testimony and with tackling strongholds. It can be done. There is victory if one does not give up.

You have been given the key to taking control of those pressing thoughts. Of the crippling effect of anxiety that has been left unchecked for far too long. It is time to pick yourself up, put on the Armor of God and learn his Truth. Walk it out every single day. Speak His truth over yourself and your situation.

It is time to start gathering the stones. Time to start

swinging your slingshot. It is more than time to take down the giant of anxiety.

Do not back down. Do not surrender. You have the Truth. You have the tools. Do not succumb to the stronghold of anxiety. Firmly grab hold of this key and know that through Him, you can overcome all things. You can be the change in medicine that you want to see.

Hold your ground.

Overcome anxiety and watch to see what the Lord will do. Unlocking the prison of anxiety is a key to freeing your mind and reviving the heart of medicine.

Get Your Hopes Up

"But those who hope in the Lord will renew their strength. They will soar on wings like eagles; they will run and not grow weary, they will walk and not be faint."
Isaiah 40:31 *NIV*

There is an epidemic of hopelessness right now. It doesn't take much discernment to look around you and to read people's faces. Many have been hurt, and many feel lost. They have lost hope.

Listen to them. Take the time to truly hear what they are saying. When they are honest, many feel that their best season is behind them. They are thinking, *"What good could possibly lay ahead right now?"*

When people are looking around for answers and solutions, they have lost their footing. They are standing on shaky ground. On sand that is crumbling beneath them. When they are given a new diagnosis or are confused as to what is going on in their mind or body, their world is in a state of upheaval.

You must not be short with them. You must be constant. You must take a moment and remember this key.

Your patients are seeking Hope. Don't get me wrong. They need medical care. But even more than this, they need hope. You need hope to help care for them.

They are coming to you for help, coming to you to find answers for what ails them. They are trying to determine if there is hope for their future. You must remind them that there is always hope. There is always a way to see light amidst the darkness. But you may be wondering, how do you convey hope to your patients?

Well, you first have to carry hope in your own heart if you are to revive it in the hearts of others.

I have often wondered how you can be in the field of healthcare and not have a relationship with God. It seems impossible to me. How can you care for those in their darkest moments and not know the One who is love and light, who holds all the answers? It is your relationship with the Savior of the world who teaches you to have hope.

Paul is speaking to you and me today when he wrote the following words so long ago:

> *"May the God of hope fill you with all joy and peace as you trust in him, so that you may overflow with hope by the power of the Holy Spirit."*
> Romans 15:13 *NIV*

You cannot truly have hope if you do not know the God of hope. You cannot overflow with hope unless you are overflowing with the Holy Spirit. The key to hope is knowing the One who is hope.

You may be wondering, though, how you keep your hope in such difficult circumstances. How do you keep your joy when we do what we do? Especially when we see the pain and hurt all around us. Such pain can be suffocating at times.

Cancer that comes as a thief and accidents that recklessly destroy. Patients who didn't have the expected ending to their stories. Parents that had to bury their children. Families that were left shattered after their loved one committed suicide. How do we not lose hope?

We must focus every single day on the only One who can give us hope. The only One who can give our patients hope. We must be so anchored in God's love that we are tethered without escape to our anchor. So anchored in the following verse, that we speak it over the mountains in front of us.

"For I know the plans I have for you," declares the Lord, "plans to prosper you and not to harm you, plans to give you hope and a future."
Jeremiah 29:11 *NIV*

Did you know that this verse was written by Jeremiah for the Israelites who were in Babylon captivity at the time? They didn't know it at that time, but we now know they would be in captivity for 70 years. Why did he speak one of the most comforting verses in the Bible in a time where circumstances were everything but what this verse speaks about? Why did Jeremiah speak of hope when it seemed like all hope was lost? Because the fact of the Israelites' captivity did not cancel the Truth of God's word.

Our patients' facts of their illness, their situations, their grief, and their hurt do not cancel the Truth of who God is. It does not cancel the Truth of a God who will always bring good out of all circumstances for those who love the Lord.

Truth is what sets you free. Truth is what allows you to be anchored to hope.

God's Truth is the only thing that can bring one hope in the lowest of valleys. Words are great. Loving actions and support are necessary. But it is the Truth about who God is, in his unchanging character, that is what gives you and I hope.

No matter what the diagnosis is for your patient, you can give them hope. You can share with them the Truth. You are never to speak over them words that destroy or crush them. You are never to dictate to them that they have a specific amount of time to live. You are not God. You are not the one who makes that call. Yes, there are natural circumstances and laws at play, but you also are not called to be cursing them with your words.

Speaking these word curses over them is extremely distressing and can give them a false certainty about something you truly do not know. There are times when patients have miraculously defied the odds. There are times when paralytics have gotten up and walked again. There are times when even the dead have come back to life.

So, for you to steal someone's hope by your careless words is not okay. You must remember to guard yourself against such things.

Darkness

There was a season of time when our family had three friends close to us commit suicide within a month's time. Each person who did this left a wake of sadness, turmoil, and questions for their families and loved ones. Questions of how they could have done this to us? How did we not know they were experiencing such pain? How could we have prevented their death?

These were just a few. There were many more questions that we will never know the answers to. Yet, in all of these untimely deaths, there was one constant. Hopelessness.

The only thing that could drive a person to the point of ending their time on Earth at their own hands is hopelessness. It is simple. They were lacking hope.They lost their focus.

They were focused on the waves and not the one that calms the storm. They were focused on the insurmountable odds, not the one that defies the odds. They were focused on themselves as the creation, not on the God who created them.

In their darkness and isolation, the enemy knew he had won. In the darkness, he was able to bring about just enough confusion and impulsivity to convince them to take their life. When they lost hope, the enemy struck.

This hopelessness is what we are battling. Hope is one of the keys to reviving the heart of medicine and keeping our patients and ourselves alive. We are not just battling with flesh and blood but with principalities.

"For we are not fighting against flesh-and-blood enemies, but against evil rulers and authorities of the unseen world, against

mighty powers in this dark world, and against evil spirits in the heavenly places."
Ephesians 6:12 *NLT*

The spiritual battle is just as real as the physical battle. Open your eyes and see the truth. The spiritual realm is more daunting than the physical one ever could be.

Medicine and the field of healthcare are practiced in treating flesh and blood, but we are not only stopping the bleeding in the physical realm. We are called to help our patients heal on all levels. To bandage the spiritual wounds as well. We are to remind ourselves and our patients that although we are battling against sickness and death, there is reason to still have hope.

The God of hope has overcome this world. He has overcome the enemy. The battle is already won. We have the choice to choose Him. When we do this, we have the hope of eternal life.

Eyes that Could Not See

I remember the night when I was called over to my parents' house. I remember I had just parked our car in our driveway after arriving home from an awesome day up in Medford with friends. I was tired and wanted to head to bed, yet I felt unsettled. I figured I would swing by my folks before I headed to bed. Something was telling me I should just check in and say hi. I now know Who that something was that was speaking to me to check in that night.

When I arrived next door, my dad was standing in the kitchen. He was mindlessly standing at the counter, and I could tell he was concerned. He was much quieter than normal. If you know my dad, seeing him silent was a worrisome sign. He told me that he was worried about my mom, and he wanted me to come take a look at her. He wasn't sure what was going on.

As I rounded the corner to her room, I saw she was lying on her bed. Her eyes seemed unfocused, and she was lying there, not reading a book. Hmm. She always reads at night. What was going on?

As I began asking her questions, I heard that she had significant dizziness. She looked really tired and kept blinking her eyes. I then asked her why she kept blinking, and she then said, *"I can't really see. I'm looking at a black hole in the middle of my vision."*

Now, it was my turn to be concerned. I immediately told her to get some other clothes on as I was driving her to the ED. Her symptoms of vision loss and dizziness were concerning for a posterior stroke. As I was driving her to the hospital, I phoned ahead. I called the backline of the provider's office. When the voice came on the phone, I requested, *"please prep for a code stroke. I am bringing my mom in, and I will be there in 15 minutes."*

When we arrived, the flurry of activity began. This time, I was not running the code stroke. I was the bystander. This time, I was the one providing the history for my confused mom. I watched as the neurologist came on the monitor, and I worked to relay everything I could quickly to the specialist. I knew that time mattered.

As she came back from the scanner, the emergency physician looked puzzled. The neurologist, myself and my mom had all been prepared to see evidence of a posterior stroke or an obvious blockage in the vasculature. Nothing. The MRI also confirmed this and showed nothing out of the ordinary. Yet, my mom still could not see, and the dizziness remained.

As the labs returned, we were shocked to find that she was in acute renal failure with hyperkalemia. One week prior, she had pristine lab results showing her baseline renal function. What was going on?!

As I was waiting for the hospitalist, I began working through the case in my mind. All I kept thinking about was the string of events that led us to this night. What had caused my mom's rapid decline? I knew she had recently had COVID and had been reporting some increased anxiety after this. She had normal labs and no evidence of a pulmonary embolism, aka a blood clot in her lungs.

It was then that I realized she was dealing with micro-clots. As their name suggests, these are small clots that clog up the tiny vessels in precious organs. These clots are so small that you won't see them on the scans. You will know their presence, though, as you will see their downstream effects, such as renal failure, vision loss, etc. Microclots are like looking at a ripple in a lake, knowing something caused the ripple, yet there is no concrete evidence of the rock that was skipped.

After thinking some more, I discussed my concerns about this with the hospitalist. Unfortunately, we were both worried about my mom's low hemoglobin level. We didn't want to give her a blood thinner if she happened to have a gastrointestinal bleed.

Well, that night became day, and I returned to her room to check on her. She continued to be very tired and confused. She kept nodding off as I was trying to talk to her. Her eyes remained unfocused. At that moment, I realized that I was not going to sit by and just watch my mom lose her eyesight. I wasn't going to let her not have vision. I knew that her absolute favorite thing to do is to read the Bible and read anything else that comes across her path. Having eyes that cannot see was not an option for her.

So, I walked down the hall and talked to the hospitalist. I decided to put myself out there. My mom deserves a fighting chance. The one who taught me to have faith, and to hold onto hope against all odds, needed us to fight for her. I was not going to give up on her healing.

So, I told the hospitalist my thoughts on the case. I then told him that I wanted to use my Electro-Equiscope machine that I had at my clinic. This machine uses microcurrents to dramatically reduce inflammation. I told him that I had seen it work on a patient who had a brain hemorrhage and watched with my own eyes as that patient had a rapid change in their neurological status within 4 hours of the first treatment. So, I asked the hospitalist if I could go outside protocol and treat my mom. If she had a microclot that was affecting her vision, time was of the essence. The hospital did not have this machine, but I had it available. She deserved a fighting chance. What is the harm of trying?

After giving it some thought, he said, *"Go ahead. Do the treatment. I don't have anything to offer otherwise at this time."* That was all I needed. I immediately went to grab the machine and brought it quickly back to begin the treatment. Once I hooked up all the electrodes and started the protocol, the 45-minute treatment flew by. I didn't see any change immediately, so I went home to rest for a couple of hours. I had left my mom in safe hands, with her best friend as her bedside advocate.

It was 2 hours later that I got the call from her friend. She had been sitting with my mom the whole time when suddenly my mom sat up in bed. She said she had a severe headache that had just started. She then became clear headed, was no longer somnolent and had gotten approximately 80% of her vision back. Within 2 hours of treatment, she looked like a different person. My hope was rising again.

Unfortunately, my mom's kidneys continued to decline. She was borderline needing dialysis and kept having dangerously elevated potassium levels. As we were only at a tiny hospital, we could not offer this treatment for her. As the hours went by, it looked more and more like she needed to be transferred.

Her kidneys continued to not respond to fluids or the medications she was receiving. Now, we needed an accepting hospital to possibly offer dialysis. Unfortunately, there were no beds. The hospital that she needed to be at was not accepting any transfers. How is this always the case?!

Well, I was raised better than to accept defeat. I was not going to accept this ending for my mother. I was not going to just sit and watch my mom worsen in front of me. No, she deserves the best.

I had her vitals checked and they were currently stable. As a physician, I knew she was safe to make the quick trip to the other hospital. We signed the paperwork needed, and I drove her quickly to the next hospital. My sister drove behind us the whole way. Her daughters were not giving up on her. We were not giving up hope for her to get well again.

As we drove, I remember thinking, *"I can't lose my mom.*

I can't lose the one who means everything to me. She has to make it. God, please don't let this happen." We continued the drive. As the darkness surrounded our vehicle that night, we fought back. We filled the car with worship songs. I knew the enemy was doing his best to discourage us and to wreak havoc in her body, yet I knew that my God was stronger than him. I knew that when we are scared, we worship. When we don't know what's up ahead, we worship. When we are fighting to keep our hope alive, we worship.

Worship is our weapon in moments when we are fighting to not lose hope. Worship was our weapon that dark night as we drove the Siskiyou Pass.

Well, thankfully we made it safely to the other hospital. We got her through the emergency department and admitted to the hospital. The enemy had tried his best, but God was with her.

There is no denying that the hospitalization had some bumps along the way. There were moments when we weren't sure if her kidneys would turn around. Yet, my mom was peaceful. She remained steady. She continued to hope and tell us that all would be fine.

She was right. I remember driving her back approximately one week later. The worship songs were still playing. The drive was now done in the light. Hope had overcome in her case. Hope had brought light again for our family.

Her sight had been fully restored. The ophthalmologist had agreed with the assessment. He believed she had micro-clots that had tried to steal her sight. But God had allowed the right pieces to fall into place. He had broken through for her. God was the key piece for her to have hope against all odds.

The one who taught me to have hope was now the one who had been a testimony of hope. The enemy, using sickness to come against her like a flood, could not penetrate the hedge of protection God had placed around her. His love surrounded her on all sides.

God never promised us that the weapons would not form, but if we stay close to Him, they will not prosper. We must never lose hope. Hope is our weapon for good. It is a way we can fight back against the darkness we are continually battling every day. We may not always win, but we must continue to always have hope.

It's Your Call

We have the choice to follow the One who is trustworthy and who we can place our hope in. We get to have the greatest hope of all that one day, we will see our loved ones again. One day, there will be no more death and disease. One day, we will be surrounded by the One who is Love and who is the healer of everything and everyone.

So today, remember to have hope. Remember that you carry hope for your patients. In your decisions, in your plans of care, in treatment protocols or recommendations that you give, make sure to keep this in mind.

In moments of hopelessness and despair, refocus your own gaze. Realize that God is always good. If you are not seeing something good right now, the story is not finished yet. He is in the process of working to redeem all things. Sometimes, we do not see the good on this side of eternity. But one day, we will see good. One day, we will see the new creation. We will see that death is no more and that all things are new again.

So, get your hopes up. Let your hope rise again. You may have seen many defeats, but that does not mean that victory is not coming. You may have witnessed many losses, but that does not mean you aren't part of the winning team.

Refocus your gaze on Him. Start each day in His presence. Seeking after the God of Hope. Seeking after the One who is love. Asking the Holy Spirit to fill you and restore the hope and joy of your salvation.

Set your eyes on Him and know that you and your patients can hope again. They are looking to you. Help them look to Him.

There is hope for your future. There is hope for the future of medicine. Hope is a key to reviving your heart and the heart of medicine.

Unshakeable Faith

Is anything too hard for God? Is there anything that He
cannot do? These are questions you need to become familiar
with as a friend of God. Questions that you need to firmly
know the answer to in your heart. Your answer to these questions determines what type of person you will be, how far
you will go in life, and who you will be in the lives of others.

Now let me ask you this. Have you ever believed for
something really big? Something that others thought you
were crazy to believe for. Something that defied the odds in
the natural world. Something where, unless God stepped in,
it would never happen. A situation where you put yourself
out there, believing in something you haven't yet seen,
waiting in faith for God to move.

I have. Many times. Thinking about it more, having

unshakeable faith has become a large part of my story and how I operate. Unshakeable faith moves you to act. It moves others to act. It moves God's hand.

This type of faith is why there is a book in Hebrews that is referred to as the Hall of Faith. It is found in Hebrews 11, and it is an amazing passage about the heroes of faith and the crazy things they believed God for. It lights up the path they blazed for us. It moves the hearts of those who are courageous enough to follow in their footsteps. If you haven't recently done so, I would encourage you to read it. Soak it in.

Unshakeable faith is unrelenting. It is steady. It is stubborn. It believes God to bring the rain even when you haven't seen the first cloud in the sky. Having this kind of faith is necessary if you are going to see God do unexplainable things. It is a key to fulfilling all that God calls you to be.

Unshakeable faith is a key to healing yourself and others.

Deep Roots

I come from a long line of hardcore believers. I was blessed to be raised by a mom who taught me to always believe for more. A mom who taught me to have faith in God doing the impossible. A woman who taught me to trust that He would always come through for me. He spoke to me many times through watching her gift of faith. He taught her to pass along the unshakeable faith that she had to her daughter. My life and success are a byproduct of the faith that she instilled in me.

We all need that person who speaks life into us. One who helps us to have unshakeable faith. One who is in your corner, continually telling you to keep knocking on the doors of heaven. My mom and my husband are those people to me.

I still remember my mom telling me that my father shouldn't have made it as an orthopedic surgeon. As a child, I remember not quite understanding all the implications of his health journey early in his career. I had heard stories but did not understand the gravity of what was said.

As I became a physician and began to care for my patients, the story she had shared became even more meaningful. She took me back to the time when she was a perinatal nurse educator at Loma Linda University. My mother and father were living in a house in Loma Linda, and she was pregnant with my sister. She had just been put on bed rest and was doing administrative work from home. She may have been on bed rest, but she was still acting as the backbone of the family while my father was busy completing his third year as an orthopedic resident.

That was when it happened. At a time that was least expected.

First, my father experienced vision loss. A short period of disturbance in the visual field that was quite alarming. It resolved as quickly as it had started. Then, there was an area of numbness in his upper leg. An event that had occurred two times. They were rattled. What was going on?

My father was supposed to be in the prime of his life. He was very healthy and active overall. This period was interrupted by this cluster of unrelated neurological symptoms that presented at various times. Since my father came from a medical family himself, his parents were rightfully worried when they heard these troubling symptoms. They immediately flew out to be present and support my parents.

After he went through the typical battery of tests to determine what the neurological symptoms were stemming from, they were told that he had Multiple Sclerosis. A progressive neurological disease that can significantly impair one's ability to perform many activities. They were told that there was only a 10% chance that he did not have this diagnosis, based on the findings of the cerebrospinal fluid analysis.

He was crushed. His parents were crushed. He was their long-awaited son. The only boy in the family. The one for which so many hopes and dreams rested on. In a moment, his future became murky. In a moment, their world had changed. They wondered, what lay ahead.

I remember my mom telling me that the news spread quickly. Soon, his academic advisor pulled him aside and told him he needed to reconsider his career in orthopedic surgery. He told him that, considering the diagnosis, he should switch to a specialty that was less physically demanding. He recommended he shadow a colleague in another field. That wasn't going to happen, though. Not with my mom in the picture.

She was at home on bed rest. She had heard the news that the life they had planned may look much different than they had expected. Yet, that was not the final word. In her mind, she went back through how he had unexpectedly been given this opportunity. She remembered how he had stopped his residency in general surgery when he received a call from his best friend at Loma Linda University telling him about this one open slot for the orthopedic residency.

She remembered that he had beat out very competitive candidates to land this opportunity and that he was flourishing in his new role.

She didn't accept the facts she had been told. They did not line up with the faith she held. My mom's mind was made up. Her faith was stronger than the fear. She looked back on how the hand of God had moved on their life, and she stopped. She stopped going down the worst-case scenarios route and looked at it from a new perspective. She looked through the eyes of faith.

She politely disagreed with the recommendation that had been given by the advisor. She saw the facts, but she was moved by the Truth. She believed he would be okay. She believed that the 10% chance meant that the odds were in their favor. She believed that the God she served had not moved them to this location and opened up this residency spot to have the door slammed firmly in their faces. No, this was not how God moves.

She had unshakeable faith.

My dad is now 73 years old, and he is still a practicing orthopedic surgeon. With the love, support and unshakeable faith of my mother, my dad sailed through his residency and enduring career without any further unexplained episodes.

Did that mean there were no other bumps along the way? Absolutely not. Yet, the fear was not allowed to stop his purpose. Faith was needed to overcome the attacks of the enemy.

You must remember this in your own life. You will always have the chance to choose faith over fear. It's your call. Your results will be influenced by your mind and soul. The enemy is always waiting, trying to plant doubts.

We must hear the voice of God louder than the enemy's taunts.

What would my dad's career have looked like if he would have settled for that first opinion? If my parents would have just accepted the recommendation to switch careers. What would my dad's life have been like if he did not have the right woman by his side?

Your choices matter. Who you allow yourself to be influenced by can shift your entire life. The thoughts you think and the words you speak can either help you reach your potential, or they can pull you off course.

Do you think that the enemy did not want my dad to have the impact he has had in the decades long career that he has succeeded at? Do you think that the enemy is currently telling you lies and half-truths so that you do not reach your full potential? Absolutely. Without a doubt.

Take inventory of who is currently speaking into your life. You must realize how powerful thoughts and words are. Things must always happen in the spiritual realm before you see them manifested physically. Actions cannot occur without the thoughts that precede them.

Remember, the enemy will always attack the seed. He will always strike in the early stages. This is why he tries to abort babies to this day. Why he tried to kill Moses before he grew up to be a deliverer of the Israelites. Why he tried to kill Jesus before he could save the world. He tries to attack at the most vulnerable stage to increase his chances of destruction and chaos.

The enemy is not stupid. He knows you have treasure inside of you. He knows that God can use you greatly if you open your mind and heart to the Lord. He knows that you hold solutions to the problems surrounding you. He is working daily to deceive you and strip the authority that you hold. If he can convince you to focus only on the fear, he can abort your purpose in life.

You are part of the Great Controversy. You are a treasure that is being fought over. You are priceless. One does not fight over useless trash. You must realize you have immeasurable value.

Yet, you must allow faith to water the seed in your life. It is faith that is needed if you are going to see mountains moved out of the way. It is unshakeable faith that is needed for you to become all you were created to be.

Confessions of a Beauty School Dropout

There are going to be times in life when you are given a word that defies reasoning and logic. A word from God that asks you to believe for fruit before you have even seen the seed.

This has been one consistent truth I have experienced in my walk with Him. He has always asked me to trust Him and have faith before I see my dreams come to pass. He gives me the next step in front of me but does not light up the whole path. He walks with you but you must always be looking to Him for your next steps. This is why it is said He is a lamp unto my feet. Not a headlight. Not a streetlight or even a spotlight. A lamp.

My guess is that He does the same thing with you. He has not given you the blueprints for every aspect of your life. Yet, His fingerprints are all around you. His love surrounds and inspires you.

Ask yourself. What dreams has He placed on your heart? What promises are you waiting for? What circumstances is He asking you to step out in unshakeable faith for?

I will let you in on a few of my own. For starters, my whole medical career has been a faith journey. My walk to get to where I am today was not a straight route. Definitely not. There were many twists and turns along the way. My journey to becoming a physician actually started with me being a beauty school dropout. Yes, you read that correctly.

After high school, I signed up for cosmetology school. I went from being a salutatorian in my high school class to dropping out of "*beauty school*" after 1 week. How did that happen? The quick answer is that I rapidly learned it wasn't for me.

I still remember walking in the first day to that cosmetology school in Medford, OR and knowing something was seriously wrong. I had enjoyed doing nails on myself and my friends and simply thought that was what I would do with my life. That was until I walked in that day to class. Immediately, I knew deep down I wasn't supposed to be there. I knew it wasn't for me. In a moment, I could see my future, but this was not it.

Have you ever had that feeling? That pit in your stomach that you were not where you were supposed to be? Well, I had it that day, and it hit me like a ton of bricks. This is not to be offensive to anyone in the beauty industry. Absolutely not. I very much appreciate those who are gifted in the field. I am just not one of them. It was not my calling to do this work.

Well, that week passed like a kidney stone. Soon, my parents got over the shock of their daughter being a *"beauty school dropout."* I wish I could say this excused me from having to hear the song from Grease being played, joyously taunting my failure at my stalled career choice. That would not be truthful, though. I have heard it several times since.

It was then, though, that I decided I was going to go to college. It wasn't long after this *"failure"* when I began working on my second career option. I had decided hair and nails were out. Chemistry and biology were in. So, I decided I would become a physician.

Medicine was My Plan B.

Looking back on this, I now laugh. It cracks me up that I was so blind to the path God had laid before me. How many times do we try to blaze our own path and miss what is right in front of us all along? How many clues and cookie crumbs must God place on our path?

Well, each class I took in college was a stepping stone. Each time I passed a test and did well in a class, I remember thinking that I was one step closer to my goal. I remember getting through organic chemistry and knowing that if God could help me get through that class, He would break open the doors for me becoming a physician.

It was then that an academic advisor stepped in. It was subtle at first, almost imperceptible. Yet, the lies of the enemy were starting to hiss. I was at the end of my time at SOU, applying for medical school, and I had it on my heart that I was going to go to Loma Linda University School of Medicine. It didn't make sense, but I just had faith that I was going to make the admissions cut and get in. I didn't want to apply to many medical schools. I figured I would just apply to three.

Yes, I know. It wasn't the "*wise choice*" when looking at it from a worldly perspective, but I was a broke student who didn't want to spend money applying to lots of programs. I figured I really only wanted to go to that one. So, my advisor gave it to me straight. He said bluntly that I was not going to get into medical school. He told me I needed to change my application process and expand my reach. If not, he promised I would not become a physician.

Well, he didn't realize he was dealing with someone with stubborn faith. He didn't realize I had Eastman blood in my veins and didn't realize that I had been raised for this fight. I heard the words coming out of his mouth, but they didn't register. They didn't break my faith.

Well, he ended up being wrong in his assessment. If I remember correctly, I was the only one that year that matched into an MD program. God had given me a word, and I knew deep down that He would fulfill His word. In the natural, I looked like I was lacking wisdom. In His realm, I was just walking the path He had for me.

That is the thing with stubborn faith. You must be on guard and realize the enemy will send people to discourage you. He will send those to try to dig up the seed before it becomes fruit. It is your job to know when it is God speaking and when you are hearing the lies of the enemy.

This is why your relationship with Him matters. You must know His voice. You must know His character. You cannot trust if you don't know the One you are putting your trust in.

You must learn to hear the Word of God above the noise.

His voice will drown out the taunts of the enemy and allow you to have unshakeable faith.

Promised to Multiply

I am going to let you in on something that is very personal. A part of my story that cuts deep, yet is an important part of my journey to help others. I am currently standing in faith for a much larger promise. One that is bigger than my calling in medicine. One that is the calling to be a mother.

I didn't realize how much I wanted to have children until I met my husband. The first day that I met Jason, I came home and told my family and friends that I would marry him. Yes, they gave the same look that you now have. They thought I was crazy.

Jason and I had begun chatting online for a few months before I met him in person. I remember thinking he was too good to be true, and I was worried that I would be let down when I met him in person. That couldn't have been further from the truth.

The night before I met Jason in person, I remember writing in my journal that tomorrow would be *"the day I saw God's divine blessings."* I couldn't explain it. It was a certainty. I knew deep down in my spirit that something would shift the day I met him. This was exactly what happened.

The first day we met, I began seeing life in a different way. It was as if all of the hurt and pain from my past no longer mattered. I remember looking at him and knowing that it was going to be okay. It was all worth it. Every part of my journey had prepared me for him.

In a moment, your life can change. In a moment, someone can come across your path that forever changes your story. We must always be open to these divine interruptions.

For me, the first day with Jason, my life forever changed. I knew that God had brought us together and had amazing plans for us. Thankfully, he felt the same. We were engaged a few months after that. He took me to the top of Table Rock Mountain, the place he had taken me on our first date. What had felt like an eternity to find each other was now just a blip in time. We had found our forever person in each other.

With our storybook romance and the love we had found, I just knew that we would have children right away. I had loved becoming a stepmom to our daughter Gracie, but I longed for biological children. I longed to experience this chapter of life together.

Well, the days turned to weeks. Months turned to years. Each month, I was devastated by the lack of pregnancy. Each month, my world was growing darker.

For many of the years, I was still working in the Emergency Department. I remember how my heart would break each time I told a mother the exciting news that she was expecting. It was often further broken by the mothers who were devastated by that news. Carrying joyful news to someone who viewed it as an inconvenience truly broke me. There were many nights that my husband had to physically pick me up off the ground. He tried to bring comfort in a situation where I could not be comforted.

Well, as the years went by, we continued to believe for

our children. We had a knowing deep down that we would have twin girls. We had people who didn't even know us come up and prophesy to us about our children. We had people who were prayer warriors tell us that God had been speaking to them about continuing to pray for our babies. Yet, they still did not come.

It was eight years after we met that I turned 40. Eight years of hoping and praying for a breakthrough in a barren wilderness. Eight years that felt like 40. Yet, I continued to seek God. I continued to hear His loving voice. I continued to hear Him say, *"Focus on caring for my children. Focus on caring for those I bring across your path, and I will bring you your children."*

I will not go into all of the details of this chapter in my life because I know it will be written about later, but I will say a couple more things. I remember going to a women's conference in the spring of 2024. I had shown up alone. I had gone with no expectations other than to spend time with my God. To radically experience Him and His love. Deep down, I knew there was a word for me at that conference.

It was at the end of the first night that I remember going forward for an altar call to the front of the room. Alex Seeley had been preaching, and she had asked mothers to come up to the front of the room. In faith, I remember going up to the front of the room for prayer. I knew I was a mother to Gracie, but in my heart, I was still longing for my other children.

That night, things began to shift in the most amazing of ways. The hurt began to fade away. I knew I was in a moment that was shifting the ground beneath me. One of those times where the fault lines were shifting. I remember there was a point when Alex was asking for people to raise their hands if they were dealing with a certain issue. Some with trauma from broken mother relationships and old wounds. Some had children who had gone off track and were in the grip of addiction. Neither of these were me. I just listened and waited for my moment.

At the final moment, the eleventh hour, my world shook. It was her final prayer that was directed straight at my heart. She ended the altar call that night with women who wanted to become mothers. Those dealing with the desolate journey of barrenness. She was going after my deepest wound. The area in my life where it hurt me the most to stand in faith for. The one that had cost me endless sleepless nights and had, at times, me questioning God's love and faithfulness for me.

Yes, deep wounds bring up the most difficult questions. Yet, these are the dark places where His light shines the brightest. These are the areas where scars form and slowly stop our hearts from beating. We must not keep these parts from Him. We must let Him into these dark places if He is going to light them up. We must let the ultimate Surgeon cut away the scar tissue if we are going to have our hearts revived again.

That night, I still remember dropping to the ground when I heard the call for prayer for this. I remember ugly crying, like Hannah in 1 Samuel, as my heart broke for a promise not yet fulfilled. It was at this moment that many women surrounded me. I still remember being enveloped by an overwhelming feeling of love by women who I did not know.

As I was praying at this moment, suddenly, there was someone speaking in my ear. I leaned in closely, trying to hear what they were saying. They kept repeating a phrase over and over. I shut out all the noise and listened harder. What were they saying? I then heard it for the first time. The words *"It's not a matter of if, but when. It's not a matter of if, but when."* It was then that I opened my eyes. Then, that I looked at the face of the person who was speaking these healing words to me. Words that my spirit fully agreed with.

Gasp. It was Alex Seeley, herself!

I hadn't realized it since my eyes had been closed and blurry from all the tears but she had gotten off the stage to come and pray for me. To take the time to speak words of encouragement. Words of life that came into my soul and were an anchor to my promise. She was replacing the lies of the enemy with the words of God.

In a moment, my hope began to rise again. In a moment, I realized that what I thought I had given up on had not been forgotten by God. He sees me. I know He sees you too.

That night, He sent His friend to me. A person who had battled infertility herself, to come to comfort another one of His children. He had broken through the veil for me. He remembered me. He was still speaking His love and promises over my life.

I didn't know it could get better after that, but the next night blew my mind once again. As I was sitting in my seat, a woman next to me handed me a golden necklace. One that had the number 11:24 written on it. A beautiful necklace with colon marks made of two diamonds. I looked at the gift in disbelief. *"Why are you giving this to me?"*

She took a breath and told me the story. She said she

had been at a store approximately 8 months prior, and she had seen the necklace. The sparkle had caught her eye. She said that God told her she was to get the necklace. She questioned Him about it. She said that she never wore necklaces, and she asked Him, "*Why am I to get this necklace?*". He told her that it was not for her, but He would reveal to her, at the right time, who she was to give the necklace to.

She was faithful and picked up the necklace. She kept the necklace for many months before she heard His next instructions. She said that morning, when she got up to come to the conference, she heard Him clearly speak again. This time, He told her to put on the necklace. He told her that today was the day she would give it away, and He would reveal to her who she would give it to.

She went on. She said, "*When you sat down, He told me the necklace was for you.*"

I was shocked. I asked what it all meant. What were the numbers written on the necklace? She told me they were in reference to a verse in Mark. The numbers were speaking the Word of God to me,

"Therefore I tell you, whatever you ask for in prayer, believe that you have received it, and it will be yours."
Mark 11:24 *NIV*

She was speaking to me about the promises of God in my life. She was speaking to me about the children I had been promised. With that golden necklace, she literally gave me the gift of faith.

That night, God worked through one of His friends to send me a message. He knew how much I needed this gift. He gave me His promise to wear directly over my heart. A visual representation of His abundant love for me. I realized I may be waiting on promises to come into the physical realm, but I have the God of the universe who is carrying me in my waiting.

If you have not directly experienced His gifts to you, don't despair. Keep looking. Keep seeking after Him. Desire Him with your whole heart and He will give you the desires of your heart. He will send people across your path who breathe life back into your weary soul. It may take time, but His promises are never truly delayed. They are in His timing.

Well, it was after this conference that I began to see the path light up before me. I began to truly believe that, even with God's long-awaited promises, they are Yes and Amen.

I still claim this promise. I still look to Him to fulfill His word to me. I know that it's not a matter of if but when.

That is the thing about unshakeable faith. God doesn't ask you to have it alone. He doesn't ask you to have faith without knowing He is faithful. He is walking right beside you. He will pick you up and carry you when you fall. Unshakeable faith was always meant to grow in community. Amidst other believers who would be keys to your promises fulfilled. To stand with you in faith to move mountains.

What mountains in your life need to be moved? Sometimes these mountains move one pebble at a time. Don't give up if you do not see things shift the first time you pray. What promises are yet to be fulfilled in your life? You must realize that He is the God who fulfills His word. You must see your promises in your heart before you hold them in your arms.

Your patients are the same as you and me. Others around you are just as desperate in their waiting rooms of life. They need your gift of faith. They need your words of Truth. They need encouragement when they fall down. Lift them up by your words. Carry them when they can no longer carry themselves.

Your coworkers need you to walk alongside them and hold up their arms when they are feeling weak. You cannot win battles alone. It is going to take a team working together to accomplish great feats. You must refocus their gaze beyond the current challenges and help them see a brighter future.

Your family needs you to speak Life to them. To love them into wholeness and continually lift them up. To redirect their gaze when they are drifting in their faith.

God is waiting for you today. He has great plans for you. He is faithful. He can be trusted. Have the faith to step forward today, knowing that He will be the one to catch you when you fall. Know that He is walking there right beside you.

Remember, if He has spoken a Word to you, He will be faithful to His Word. If He has put a promise on your heart, it's not a matter of if but when it will show up.

Faith is a key to reviving your heart with the promises of God. Faith is the key to walking into your next chapter. Faith is a key to reviving the heart of medicine.

THE FINAL HOUR

"The Lord is my shepherd; I shall not want. He makes me lie down in green pastures. He leads me beside still waters. He restores my soul. He leads me in paths of righteousness for his name's sake. Even though I walk through the valley of the shadow of death, I will fear no evil, for you are with me; your rod and your staff, they comfort me. You prepare a table before me in the presence of my enemies; you anoint my head with oil; my cup overflows. Surely goodness and mercy shall follow me all the days of my life."
Psalm 23:1-6 *ESV*

There are times when God does His greatest work in our final hours. Times when we witness the true shifting of a spiritual atmosphere. The moments where God comes especially near to one of His closest friends.

As those in the field of medicine, it is an honor and a privilege to be the ones that advocate for our patients in these moments. In the moments when our patients' time on

Earth is growing short. What we often don't realize, though, is that we are witnessing something much bigger than we imagined. Something that is more important than anything in this physical realm. It is these times that are to be cherished.

In these hours, we are watching God do His most important work in the spiritual realm. We are witnessing Heaven invade Earth, seeing healing on the spiritual level. We do not understand all of God's ways. We never will when we are living on Earth. God is sovereign. Yet, one day we will understand.

There are times when God's answer does not line up with what we would choose. Yet, He always brings the full picture together, all in His timing. All in love. This does not mean there is no pain that is part of this process, or even heartache. Don't stop running to Him when you are hurt. Keep seeking Him even in your pain. I promise you, God will redeem it. He will use all things for His glory and to bring healing on all levels.

So, I am going to take you on one last journey of our God working in unusual ways in a patient's final hours. Take your shoes off and get comfortable. You are about to learn of the final hours of one of my most cherished friends. One of God's friends.

This story speaks of one of my most beloved patients. The pastor who baptized me when I was a young teenager. The one who originally showed me the picture of the true Advocate, the Holy Spirit.

To know Pastor Sam was to love him. You could not help but be drawn in by his warm smile. Everyone who came across his path shifted closer to him. They could not help but be transformed by being near him.

When you were with Sam, you could not help but feel the presence of his Friend all over him. He was filled with the love of God. He exuded peace in any space that he walked into.

Knowing Sam meant knowing the love of the Father. He was the ultimate in shifting atmospheres. I have never met anyone like him or his wife in all the years I have done patient care. They will always hold that spot in my heart. That was why it was so devastating when I heard the news.

I still remember standing in my living room when I heard his wife on the phone, her voice cracking as she shared that they had just learned Sam had an advanced stage of cancer. It was like clouds covering the sun. The atmosphere immediately darkened. The room felt stuffy. A weight pressed down on me. I listened carefully as she explained what the diagnosis was and the information they had been given.

I did not accept it. I did not accept that we were just going to sit by and watch Sam leave us without fighting against this terrible disease. So, I didn't. I pleaded with God. I asked that He would give us answers. Give us more time.

God began speaking to me. He began waking me up at night with messages. Messages to send to His friend. Messages of encouragement. Messages of hope.

On the day that Sam was being anointed by the elders in his church, I was up in my bedroom. I could not travel to this event as he did not live in the same town. That day, though, I was putting away clothes when I heard the familiar voice of my friend, the Holy Spirit. It was clear. Very short, but clear. *"Pray for my servant Samuel."* That's all I heard. I immediately stopped putting away clothes and began to pray for my friend. For God's friend.

It was not long after this, He had me send a message to Sam. This message included the exact words God had spoken to me. These words were to remind His friend that he was, *"My servant Samuel"*. Even in the pain, God was speaking Sam's true identity over him. He was not allowing the arrows from the enemy to have the final say.

I did not know it at that time, but this exact message was given to Sam as a child. These were the words God spoke to Sam when He first called him into the ministry. That is the thing with words of knowledge. God uses them to get our attention. He uses them to wake others up. Listen carefully when God speaks to you. You never know how He is wanting to work through you.

Well, this specific message started Sam and I on the next steps of his journey. It wasn't long before he decided to come up to see what could be done. To come to The Well.

When I heard that he and Sue were going to be coming up for a visit to discuss further options, I began to get our guest room ready. I remember being upstairs, making his bed and fluffing the pillows when God showed me a flashback. As they say, a picture is worth a thousand words. In the blink of an eye, He took me back to the whole reason we had prepared a guest room during the Pandemic. The start of this moment.

He took me back to a message that we had watched that had prompted my husband and me to get a guest room ready. It was a sermon given during the early days of the

Pandemic. It was during this dark night of our souls that God used another pastor's words to wake us up.

He used one living in North Carolina to speak directly into our situation in our tiny town in northern California. One whose words pierced our hearts and shifted the atmosphere in our living room that night. It was the messages that we heard from this pastor and his team that gave us hope and courage to get through this very dark time.

That's the thing about messages. You never know how your words can be used to heal or to harm. You don't have to be standing in a church to allow your heart to be revived. Sometimes, you may just be in your pajamas ugly crying on a couch. It's all the same to God. He is always after your heart.

Well, at that time, we weren't just battling the darkness of the pandemic. As an emergency medicine physician, it was arguably the darkest moment of my career. The only way I was keeping my head above water was to flood my mind with God messages. I welcomed anything I could watch to shift my attention from the darkness I was experiencing on a daily basis. Yet, it was more than that I was battling.

My husband and I had struggled with infertility for 4 years at that point. We had hoped we would have a baby room by now that was filled with love and laughter, yet this had not yet come to pass. The years had gone by, and the room remained silent. Yet, it only took one night to begin to shift our focus. A *"suddenly"* moment was about to break out.

It was while watching the sermon *"Just the 2 of Us"* that our own story began to shift. We listened intently as we heard the story of the Shunamite woman and Elisha come to life. Let me tell you. It was fire. It discussed the story in 1 Kings 4:8 where the infertile Shunamite woman prepared a room for the prophet Elisha.

This Shunamite woman was one who had never had a child, but she didn't let that stop her from serving God. She wanted to support the work of one who was called by God. She wanted to show love to one of God's children during her waiting period, even after she had lost hope in her own miracle.

She had money, and she had a heart for God. So, she took her resources and created a room for the prophet to stay at. This room was available any time that he came through her town. It was this room that Elisha stayed in that eventually held her breakthrough. That eventually held the prophet who would tell her a message that shook her world. A message that said, "...*About this time next year, you will be holding a son.*"

Well, this sermon got our attention. We turned off the television and immediately made plans to create a guest room. We put what we heard into action. Over the next week, my husband used his skills as a contractor and created the perfect cozy room. I used my decorating skills and added the finishing touches. I found all the perfect pieces and made sure it had all the details I wanted.

Then we waited. We eagerly anticipated how God would use our upper room. We wondered who God would send to us so we could bless them with a space we had created ahead of time. It was a small act of obedience but one that I am forever glad we did.

That's the thing with making room. We must clear out space for God to work. We must open our hearts and our homes to what He wants to use them for. We must do our part. We must be obedient when He places something on our heart. Heaven watches to see how we respond when our heart is stirred.

The flashback ended as quickly as it had begun. I was snapped right back to reality.

It had taken some time but God was revealing to me why He had told us to create a room in advance. Three years before His friend Samuel would need it. This shows how special Sam was.

That is the thing with God and His messages. They often do not happen right away. He gives us directions that we are to follow and then we wait on Him and His timing. We must be faithful in stewarding what He told us. We must quickly respond in faith if we are going to be usable by Him. We must not give up in our waiting period. It may take some time but God is never late.

Well, that day, I did not say a word about this sermon to anyone as I continued to get the room ready. I pondered what God was doing with all of this. What was He up to? Why did He show me this flashback?

Well, Sam and Sue arrived, and I was beyond happy to see my friends. Although the circumstances were not desirable, I was doing everything I could to soak in time with them. We all went to bed that first night. We were ready for some rest. I had not shared anything with Sam and Sue about their room. I just prayed that night that they would find peace and comfort while staying with us. I also prayed for supernatural healing and insight into his case.

The next day, Sam walked down the stairs. You could hear his footsteps slowly coming down the stairs. You could tell he was in pain, but he gently came down the stairs and made his way into the kitchen. As he sat there, he had a brightness in his face. He was smiling.

You could tell he was about to share something that had piqued his interest. He went on to tell me what had happened that night. The night that he first slept in our upper room.

He said, *"I woke up around 1 am this morning. It was very interesting. God woke me up with a story in the Bible. He was speaking to me of a very specific Bible verse. Do you know of it? Have you heard of 1 Kings 4:8? It is the story of the Shunamite woman and Elisha. On her preparing the upper room for the prophet."*

He went on.... *"I mean, I know I am not a prophet, but it seems uncanny that you prepared an upper room for me that I am now staying in. It reminds me of that story."*

Wow! My jaw about hit the counter. Now, it was time for me to be shocked.

It was then that I told Sam about the beginnings of his upper room and the story of how it came to be. I told him that he was indeed staying in an upper room that God had told us to prepare for someone He would be sending to us. Sam was that person. Sam was the Gift that God sent to me. An Advocate. A prophet. A friend of God.

That was the start of the end of his time on Earth. The beginning of Sam's journey back in Yreka included a supernatural encounter where God was speaking to His friend Sam as well as to me. He was bringing our stories together. He was weaving together pieces of His tapestry. He was showing that He was here with us, even in this dark hour.

There is more to healing than just the physical, though.

God is always after true healing of one's heart and soul. He is not focused on superficials.

Well, there are too many things to speak of that occurred in the next few months, but it was a period of many visits for my friend. It was a time of so many things that we were trying to help Sam with physically and that other providers were doing their best to help him with as well.

There were people that God was directly placing in Sam's path, and He was being a gift to them. He was helping others as he was going through his own health journey. That's how special Sam was. He truly had a heart of gold. He had the heart of the Father.

Sam would shift the atmosphere at any clinic or hospital he walked into. Everyone who came near Him experienced the love of God. Every time you were near Sam, you never felt like you had enough time with him. One day with Sam was better than so many days not in his presence. His heart made you hunger for the heart of God.

Not only was Sam helping others in his darkest hours, God was still working on Sam. He was still refining him in the fire. He was bringing any of the tiniest impurities to the surface so that He could shine even brighter for Him. God was encountering His friend in stronger ways than he said he had experienced in the many amazing years of his ministry.

That's the thing with God. He creates masterpieces and continues to shape and mold us. Yet, we must submit ourselves to the Potter's wheel. In His hands, we can reflect His love more strongly each and every day. If we let Him work long enough on our hearts, we can become true vessels of His glory. Sam knew this truth. His life reflected this. He had spent time with the Potter and he was greatly refined.

I still remember Sam being at The Well when he spoke the words I never thought he would say. He said, "*I can't believe I'm saying this, but I am thankful for the cancer. I am thankful for this journey. I didn't realize it before, but this journey has allowed me to know God in a completely different way. I have walked others through their dark hours and struggles with cancer, but now God is walking me through this. He is revealing himself in ways I didn't know before.*" It was as if Sam was quoting Job when he said,

"*My ears had heard of you but now my eyes have seen you.*"
Job 42:5 *NIV*

Sam's words shifted my priorities that day. They shook my world. I had never heard a patient say something so profound. I had never witnessed God speak so clearly through a patient.

I should've realized that this was how God works. That one of His closest friends would impart a message that would impact me to this day. A message that would change how I would look at battles that I was facing on a daily basis with my other cancer patients. Sam's words still echo in my heart today.

I didn't know it then, but time was growing short for him. He was not long for this world. The time flew by much too quickly. It was not long before I got another phone call. A call from his family that Sam was not doing well. Another shift was coming.

When I heard the description of how he was and what his vitals were, I cancelled my other patients and immediately drove down to that small Emergency Department in his hometown. I knew that this time mattered. That this was where I was supposed to be. I needed to be with my friend and his family at this moment.

Unfortunately, it was not a time that you can ever prepare for as a friend. These are the kind of moments that you never forget. As a physician, yes, you know how to go through the motions. But as a friend, it is much different. As a friend, you are crushed to walk with them in this hour.

As we heard the news of how his systems were all shutting down, the only thing I could think of was that I was blessed to have known him. Blessed to have been part of this journey for my friend. I was crushed, but I was blessed.

As the doctor was telling him the horrible news, Sam was peacefully saying, *"God, you are so good. God, you are so good."* I will never forget those words as he spoke them. They were the words of a true friend of God. His countenance reflected this truth. His body was failing him, yet his spirit was growing stronger in the Lord.

His words that day showed that he trusted his Friend and knew He was good, even when the news was not good. His words impacted even the young physician who was caring for him in that emergency department. I am sure of it.

It was not much longer after that when my friend was peacefully laid to rest. When I spoke with Sue, she said he was very comfortable and had a peaceful time enjoying the love of his family those last few days. God had allowed His friend to not suffer in his final moments. I believe it is because Sam was so full of God's love that the darkness had no choice but to flee.

Sickness may have won the battle that day, but we all

know that God has already won the war. Soon, death will be no more.

Was I heartbroken? Yes. Was I upset with God's answer that he had not healed him? Yes. But then I thought back to a conversation Sam and I had. God reminded me of a conversation where Sam had told me that he was wanting to stay alive long enough to see the outpouring of the Holy Spirit. Sam wanted to see his Friend move. He wanted to see his Friend in all His glory.

The amazing thing was God answered His friend's desire of his heart. He encountered Sam. In his final visit to our house, Sam had a life changing encounter in our upper room. He encountered God in a space that we later realized had been created just for him. During the encounter, God spoke to him and revealed a portion of His glory.

God had not let his friend down. Not even close. God came through in his final hours. He was with Sam. He showed him who He was. He poured out His Spirit on Sam and met him, even in his darkest of moments.

So, as I drove home that day from the hospital, I thanked God. I realized that we don't always get the answer that we seek, but we get to worship a God that is all loving and always amazing. A God that comes near to His friends. A God that is not distant. One that is desiring intimacy and friendship with those who are open to walking with Him. He always allows us to make a choice. We must choose to love Him. We must choose to open our hearts to Him.

Now it is your turn. Do not let disappointment be the end of your story. You may feel broken right now. You may have lost someone that is close to you. That is not the end. God is still working.

You have the chance to partner with the Holy Spirit and encounter Him in ways you never thought possible. You have the chance to hear from God when He speaks to you about His friends. You have the opportunity to experience God in His glory and to reveal it to others.

God still speaks today. He still moves today. Your greatest Friend still encounters you today. You must be willing to seek Him, though. You must be willing to open yourself up to seeing Him move in spectacular ways.

God is pouring out His Spirit right now. You must have eyes to see and ears to hear, or you will miss it. God is shifting the atmosphere of medicine right now. He wants you to be part of it. Are you willing to partner with Him and be an Advocate for others? Are you ready to see the Holy Spirit do what you never thought He could do in your life and the lives of others?

Get ready to move forward with a new wind at your back. Get ready to watch Him move. Wait and see what He can do when you surrender to Him.

Midnight hours remind us all that we are never alone. We have One who walks with us. We have One who loves us more than we can fathom. Do not let these midnight hours fool you. He is still working. We must do our part, though. We must make room for Him to move.

Midnight hours are the ones where God's light shines the brightest. In your pain, don't turn your eyes from Him. Lean in. Allow His love during your darkest moments to revive your heart once again.

BEGIN AGAIN

Have you ever resuscitated a person? Have you ever provided life giving CPR to help a heart start to beat again and oxygen enter the lungs? Have you seen someone return from the brink of death? I have.

It is not easy work. It requires a team. It requires many working in unison. All with hearts and minds focused on one thing: the patient and the monitor. Looking to see the heartbeat. Looking to see a flutter, a disruption of asystole on the monitor.

We do our work, and then we do a pulse check. We look to see that first heartbeat on that monitor. We see the movement. We then wait to see what damage has been done. We wait to see what our efforts of the resuscitation produced.

It is no different in the work we are called to in our daily lives. We work with all our hearts on the tasks set before us. We intervene. We act. We hope. We watch as things come to life in front of us.

Our Challenge

You and I are going to have to work with all our hearts and strength to revive the heart of medicine. To reset the paths of those around us. It is going to take the supernatural to breathe life again into this field. A field that has grown dry and cracked from division and lack of empathy and compassion. A field that has become polluted with pride and unbelief. One where patients and their healthcare teams are often not on the same page.

It is not enough, though, to just hope that medicine will improve. To wish that the field would be filled with empathy and compassion again. To wait and hope that someone else will come along and do this for us. No. It is going to take both you and me.

By now, you know that the field of medicine needs a reset. The heart of medicine must be revived. Patients need to know that there is hope again. They need to feel safe and truly cared for. You need to know you can hope again. Your colleagues need to know that you are on the same team again.

I believe it will happen. I believe there is still hope. I believe that the heart of medicine will beat again.

Begin Again

No matter how broken or seemingly beyond repair something is in this natural world, there is always time to begin again. If you are still living and breathing, today is your chance at a new beginning.

Our God is not a God of disorder. He is the God of redemption. His work is always focused on complete restoration. He does not settle for mediocrity. He does not play it safe. He does not leave us in the ruins. Yet, God's timing is not always the same as our timing. He does not always work in the early hours of our problems. He allows time for us to mature. He often waits to see how we will respond to the challenges in front of us.

Often, He seems to do his best work at 11:59 pm; A time that often seems late in our eyes. A time that almost feels hopeless. Here is the thing. He is the God of hope. He is the one who can revive any situation. There is nothing He cannot redeem. As hard as His timing is to understand, God functions outside of the realm of time. His timing on Earth may seem delayed from our perspective, but from His perspective, the timing is always perfect. He operates in eternity and has solutions that we cannot fathom.

Your situation. Your career. Your relationships. The field of medicine. There is nothing too hard for Him. There is still hope to begin again.

Full restoration is what is needed. There is a way to get to the other side. Yet, to get to the other side, we cannot continue doing the same things day in and day out and hope for a different result. We are going to need to come up higher. To be seeking after heavenly solutions.

We need a reset. We need to begin again.

Vision Precedes Provision

We have a great challenge ahead of us, but that does not mean it cannot be done. With God, the odds are always in our favor.

You may be staring right now at a massive amount of debt. Perhaps you have been blindsided by betrayal. Maybe you are burned out with your career. Or maybe you are sick and tired of healthcare professionals who keep dismissing you and your condition. The challenges may differ, yet the solution remains the same.

If you are facing a challenge that seems beyond hope, one where the odds do not seem to be in your favor, you need to take a step back. You need to take a moment to breathe. I invite you to come up higher and view it from Heaven's perspective.

"Where there is no vision, the people perish: but he that keepeth the law, happy is he."
Proverbs 29:18*KJV*

I have heard it said that vision will always precede provision. I firmly believe this to be true. I have lived it. God never asks us to blindly follow Him without first providing vision. Without first focusing our eyes on the situation that He is asking us to come up higher in. However, it is up to us to act. We must choose what to do with our vision.

We must see with our heart the desired outcome before we can experience it in the physical realm. That is what faith is. It is knowing something will come to pass before being given the evidence of its arrival. It takes vision to fulfill the call of God on your life. It takes vision to see miracles come to pass.

We aren't supposed to keep staring at the pig pen, the mess that is surrounding us. No, we are to focus our eyes on Him and what He calls us to. We are to take our eyes off the waves and refocus them on Him. We then move forward with this new focus.

When we are faithful to what God has shown us, He will be faithful in providing the resources and the outcome to accomplish our work. God can be trusted. We have to get out of our own way. We have to assess if we are following God's plans for us or going off on our own path. We must do the deep work and truly analyze what is behind our motives.

If God has called you to complete a task, if He has put something strongly on your heart to do, there is nothing on Earth that will stop you from completing what He has set before you. If He calls you to it, you will receive everything you need to complete that work. Yet, you must not sabotage the work He has for you to do.

If He has asked you to do something, it is on His heart to accomplish that purpose on Earth at that specific time. You can choose to not follow through. You can choose to hesitate and watch the opportunity pass you by, but know that His purpose will be accomplished. He will either work through you if you are willing, or He will find someone else who is courageous enough to step forward in that calling and accomplish His purposes.

It is always a choice.

All of Heaven is backing you on this. All of Heaven is waiting with the expectation that you will fulfill what He has called you to do. If He has sent you on His mission, then He will bring the funds and resources to complete those next steps. He will light up the path before you.

This is why we call Him a lamp unto our feet. His light shines ahead of us, but it does not light up the entire path to the destination. You must be courageous enough to take that next step. You must trust in His goodness and who He is and realize that He will light up your next step as you walk the path together.

52 Days

Take a moment and turn your eyes away from your current situation. Focus on the story of Nehemiah. Focus on a time when Jerusalem's walls were torn down and in total disarray. These walls had been torn down for over half a century. Many years that must have felt like an eternity to God's children.

It was at this time that Nehemiah was burdened with a cause that was much greater than his own work. His heart became burdened for God and His people. For the capital city of his homeland. To restore walls that had been broken down and seemingly beyond repair.

The full account can be found in the book of Nehemiah. As you read it, you learn that what began as a burden on Nehemiah's heart led him to pray and fast. To seek God for answers to this issue.

It was in his obedience and his heart for this issue that God gave him favor in the king's eyes. It was supernatural favor that gave him the resources he would need to success-fully bring restoration to Jerusalem's walls. What was on

Nehemiah's heart had been placed there by the Lord himself. The bill had already been paid.

He was able to use the resources he was provided and to encourage the people on assignment to work with tools in one hand and weapons in the other hand. He needed to keep them focused on the assignment while fending off the attacks of the enemy. Not only was God with Nehemiah and the people in rebuilding the wall, but He expedited their work.

"So, we rebuilt the wall until all of it reached half its height, for the people worked with all their heart."
Nehemiah 4:6 *NIV*

God helped them complete the massive project in 52 days. What had been left in utter disarray for over half a century was restored in 52 days! That is the power of our God. That is the power of those who are transformed by His heart and who are working for His cause. God can do it quickly, but you must make the choice to begin again.

Look Again

You may be looking at a gigantic mess, but to God, it is redeemable. You may feel like you have failed everything you have tried, but God is asking for you to try one more time. Breakthrough is often the next step, just beyond when you feel the most broken.

Where you see darkness, God sees an opportunity to bring light. He specializes in bringing strength to our weaknesses. He makes up for our shortcomings.

Like Nehemiah, we have a massive assignment in front of us. We are called to shift the atmosphere around us. We are called to revive the heart of medicine. It is not going to be completed in one day or by one person. It is going to take vision. It is going to take grit. It is going to take perseverance in the face of the enemy's threats and taunts.

We cannot just sit idly by and watch as the field of medicine continues to fall into disarray. To be wholly divided and with a heart of stone.

It is more than time for God's people to wake up. We are nearing the midnight hour. It is time for an army of advocates to have their bones rattled so we wake up out of our slumber and begin to fight for a cause that is much greater than ourselves. It is not a time to stand alone in division. There is too much at stake.

We can no longer wait for someone else to take care of this. We are the body of Christ. We are His people. We are His hands and feet, and we are called to care for His people.

Being in the field of healthcare is like no other career. We have the special responsibility to help people in their greatest moments of need.

People who often would never dream of walking into a church, will walk through the doors of an Emergency Department. They will seek help when they are at their lowest moments or are in pain. They will hobble through the doors of your clinic. They will roll through the doors of your operating room. They will look to you for answers to their most pressing conditions.

Here is the thing.

You have the keys now. You are the heart of medicine. You carry the heart of God. You can be the smile to comfort them at the bedside. You can have the word of encourage-ment, the exact word of hope they need to push through another day.

You are called to lead them to the One who can revive their hearts. You are called to show them the love of God.

You are not just there to be watching and waiting for someone else to step in. You have an amazing opportunity to bring His healing to anyone who comes across your path.

By hosting His presence, they are encountering Him.

By loving them, they are experiencing the Father's love.

By you speaking to them how you want to be spoken to, you are showing them what our Savior is truly like.

By praying with or for them, you are bringing them supernatural solutions.

By having a spirit of excellence, you will provide excel-lent care for them.

By forgiving others, you will be able to host Judas at your table while still washing his feet.

By laying down your pride, you will be able to be part of an amazing team that your patient needs.

By releasing anxiety, you can step forward in your purpose.

By clinging to unshakeable faith that never gives up, you will experience things too good for eyes to see.

By walking alongside them in their midnight hours, you will bring healing while simultaneously experiencing the healing of your own heart.

By being a patient who carries the heart of God, you will have the unique opportunity to heal your healers.

By refocusing your gaze on Him, medicine can begin again.

I am Sending You for the Healing of the Nations

It is time to turn that heart of stone into one of flesh again. Revival starts with you.

There is a blueprint for future healing. There is a time and a place where healing will meet all the needs of those who seek it. It can be found and read about right now.

"In the middle of its street. On either side of the river was the tree of life, bearing twelve kinds of fruit, yielding its fruit every month; and the leaves of the tree were for the healing of the nations."
Revelation 22:2 (*AMP*)

Did you read that? Did you perceive that the tree of life was planted next to a river? Did you understand that for good fruit to prosper, it must come from roots that are well watered?

Dry and cracked ground needs water to be renewed. It must be watered if it is going to produce life. Barren places require certain ingredients. They require nutrients that transform the soil. They require a constant source of water.

Your mind, body and spirit, your career, and those who come across your path all require the same substances. They require Living Water. They require a never ending source of Life. They require deep wells.

There is a Living Well. There is water that one can obtain that is never ending. Water that not only brings life to the body but water that nourishes the mind and spirit.

There is a well of Living Water. His name is Jesus Christ. He is the key to unlocking healing. He is the One who has all the answers you seek. He has sent His Spirit to help you accomplish His works in this world.

I refer to the women I work with as the "*Women at The Well*". They are women who are going after this same source of life. They are drinking deeply of this water so they can nourish, not only themselves, but others. They are not satisfied with the current dry, cracked ground of medicine.

The Women at The Well are focused on one thing: The source of Living Water. They are focused on creating a revival in medicine. They are going after healing on all levels. Our own healing. The healing of patients. The healing of a healthcare system. The healing of nations.

The Well was named after the true and living source of water. Its name has multiple meanings. Yes, it is for wellness. Yes, it is for healthcare, but it is not just a Christian integrative wellness center. It is a watering spot. It is a place that leads others to the true source of Living Water. It is a place where people come to be refreshed so they can then go out and refresh others.

We are not alone in this focus. We know there are others. There are many with their hearts turned to the source of all life.

We are seeking to be united with others in this purpose and on this mission. We know it is going to take many people to transform the current parched landscape to one that is life-giving. It is going to take many people with hearts that beat for God to revive the heart of medicine.

Patients deserve this. You deserve this.

Come Up Higher

Your heart was created to be renewed by its life source. By the Living Water that Jesus Christ gives. Your heart beats so that it can be involved in the resuscitation of other hearts. Your heart was created to beat in synchrony with your life source.

You are called to do amazing things. You are called to bring healing to others. To use all your God-given resources to help patients find health and healing.

You do not have to be a patient that accepts only partial healing. Only partial answers. No, this is not the place where you stop and rest. You are a child of God. You have an inheritance. You deserve true healing.

You are not here on a whim. God does not make mistakes. He created you for a purpose. He has great plans for you. He has called you to reveal a part of His character to all who come across your path.

Did you know that you were designed to be living at this exact time in history? You were designed with your specific attributes to reflect Him to His people. Whether you are a patient or whether you are a provider, you are part of the solution to another person's problem. You get to be a healer regardless of your exact title.

You can choose to be harsh and unloving. A critic that causes chaos and unrest. Or you can be a patient who is kind and loving. One who transforms the clinicians from whom you seek healing. No matter what your current role is, you can be the one that opens their eyes and their heart to His message.

You can be a provider whose unusual love, wisdom and care leads your patients to the Living Water.

Eyes to See

It is time to open your eyes and see what is in front of you. To see how much others truly need the heart of God in the field of medicine. To see how much others need the heart of God to get through each and every day in this dark world.

You are that vase that is overflowing with Living Water. Everyone who bumps into you should experience a fresh outpouring of His grace in their life.

He is knocking at the door today. Are you going to keep sitting there, or are you going to get up and answer the call? Do not cover your ears. Do not close your eyes. He is right by your side but you must learn to sense Him. You must open your heart to His voice and call on your life.

You are called to revive the heart of medicine. You have the keys. You are the solution. You have a heart that beats with the love of God.

Continue seeking after God first, and He will show you what it means to be a light during these dark times.

Do not let this chance pass you by. It is your midnight hour.

Reviving the heart of medicine starts with you. It starts with encountering the One who has the power to transform every area of your life. It starts with a total transformation of your own heart first. Your heart must be revived if you are to revive others.

Once you receive who He is and drink that in, you will realize that it is His love that is able to transform the world around you. It is His love that is the light that penetrates all darkness. It is His love and His presence moving through you that is the key to reviving your own heart and the heart of medicine.

Look to Him and learn His ways. Seek Him in all that you do. Experience Him and feel your heart begin to beat again. **Know in your heart that the Lord is the true Healer. To Him be all glory.**

...“If you will listen carefully to the voice of the LORD your God and do what is right in his sight, obeying his commands and keeping all his decrees, then I will not make you suffer any of the diseases I sent on the Egyptians; for I am the LORD who heals you.”
Exodus 15:26 *NLT*